Clinical Supervision Made Easy

For Churchill Livingstone:

Commissioning Editor: Susan Young
Development Editor: Catherine Jackson
Project Manager: Pat Miller
Design: Judith Wright

Clinical Supervision Made Easy
The 3-Step Method

Els van Ooijen
MA BA (Hons) DipN DipCouns PGCE RGN RM

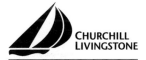

CHURCHILL
LIVINGSTONE

EDINBURGH LONDON NEW YORK OXFORD PHILADELPHIA ST LOUIS
SYDNEY TORONTO 2003

CHURCHILL LIVINGSTONE
An imprint of Elsevier Science Limited

First published 2003

ISBN 0 443 07242 6

British Library Cataloguing in Publication Data
A catalogue record for this book is available from the British Library

Library of Congress Cataloging in Publication Data
A catalog record for this book is available from the Library of Congress

Note
Medical knowledge is constantly changing. Standard safety precautions
must be followed, but as new research and clinical experience broaden
our knowledge, changes in treatment and drug therapy may become
necessary or appropriate. Readers are advised to check the most current
product information provided by the manufacturer of each drug to be
administered to verify the recommended dose, the method and duration
of administration, and contraindications. It is the responsibility of the
practitioner, relying on experience and knowledge of the patient, to
determine dosages and the best treatment for each individual patient.
Neither the Publisher nor the author assumes any liability for any injury
and/or damage to persons or property arising from this publications.

The Publisher

ELSEVIER
SCIENCE

your source for books,
journals and multimedia
in the health sciences

www.elsevierhealth.com

Coventry University

The
publisher's
policy is to use
paper manufactured
from sustainable forests

Printed in China

About the author

Els van Ooijen is a BACP (British Association of Counselling and Psychotherapy) accredited counsellor with her own consultancy, offering counselling, life coaching, supervision and training. Els has many years of experience in the health service both as a health care practitioner, trainer and lecturer. She was involved in the development of a certificate, diploma and Masters programme in (clinical) supervision for counsellors and other helping professionals at the University of Wales College, Newport where she still works as a visiting lecturer. Els has published two previous books: *Sexuality and Patient Care*, co-written with Andrew Charnock (1994), and *Clinical Supervision: A Practical Guide* (2000). As part of her ongoing personal and professional development Els is currently in the final stages of integrative psychotherapy training with the Bath Centre for Counselling and Psychotherapy.

Contents

Foreword

The unexamined life is not worth living.
(Socrates in Plato, *Apology*: 38a)

The unexamined work is not worth doing.
(Els van Ooijen, Chapter 3)

This book by Els van Ooijen presents a strong argument for all people-centred work being supported by the craft of reflective learning. This craft consists of providing the space in which counsellors can reflect on the work they have been doing and explore both the dynamics of the client and their own thoughts, feelings and behaviour. Els provides clear, practical and straightforward guidance and advice both for the practitioner and for the supervisor who enables this reflective practice.

This book builds on and develops her previous book, *Clinical Supervision: A Practical Guide*, published by Churchill Livingstone. It is rooted in her own practice both as a counsellor and as a counselling supervisor, and includes lots of personal stories and case examples. However, it is also very applicable to all others who work with people across the helping professions, whether they are therapists, teachers, social workers, doctors, nurses or other medical professionals.

The book provides an elegantly simple three-step model of supervision. Step 1 focuses on 'what': what the supervisee wants to explore; what happened in the session. Step 2 focuses on 'how': how the client session evolved; how the client and the counsellor engaged, thought and felt; the how of the dynamics. Step 3 is 'what now': how can future sessions or practice be different, based on what has been learnt from the reflective learning of this supervision session?

The craft of supervision is still quite young in its development. When Robin Shohet and I first wrote our book in the 1980s (Hawkins & Shohet 1989, 2000), there was very little published on this subject, particularly in Europe. In the USA more had been written, but mainly in the field of training clinical psychologists and focusing very much on models of the developmental stages that trainees generally progress through. Els has grounded her work very much in the British tradition, drawing together in her first chapter the various approaches of Hawkins & Shohet (1989, 2000), Inskipp & Proctor (1993, 1995), Page & Wosket (2001), Bond & Holland (1998), Carroll (1996) and Gilbert & Evans (2000). All these writers have been highly influenced by each other and in some ways form an interlinking web, network or community of thinking and practice. Indeed, there is a heartening development of reflective learning on the practice of reflective learning! Within this, the British Association of Supervision Practice and Research plays an important role. Els also cites some of the USA writers, particularly Elizabeth Holloway, who has probably done the most to link North American and European approaches.

Els' particular contribution to this stream of practice, thinking and writing is her ability to integrate and simplify many of the approaches, and to present to the new supervisor a book that is both easy to read and full of practical ways of organising their supervision. There are very good sections on how to develop a working contract, both for the supervision relationship and for a particular session, and an excellent chapter (Chapter 6) on the things that can be wrong in supervision and how to avoid these traps and pitfalls.

The last part of the book deals with the wider context of supervision, with chapters on ethics, group supervision and management, leadership and supervision in organisations.

What I most enjoyed in reading this book is the personal immediacy of Els' writing with stories such as the one that contrasts well-ordered supervision with her experience of going to the supermarket and buying something she did not want and forgetting some of the essentials! I hope you enjoy it as much as I did and that it enriches your ability to reflect on your own practice as well as to enable others to do the same.

2003   Peter Hawkins

Reviewers' comments

I am always suspicious of those who purport to make their subject 'easy' or 'simple'. Too often for 'easy' read 'very basic and introductory', or for 'simple' substitute 'simplistic'. It has been suggested that the royal route to understanding is through three stages: simplistic, complex and simple. Simple, in this context, is the end result of a long journey of search, research, reading, experience, making sense of and usually, teaching. Not many have the gift or the skill of creating 'simple' in this sense. One who does is Els van Ooijen, and this new book is an example of the kind of 'made easy' that is the culmination of a complex and lengthy scholarship.

Clinical Supervision Made Easy combines theory, research, examples, self-disclosure, transcripts, cases, practice, models, frameworks, discussions, reflection points, all woven together into an understandable, practical and highly readable book. van Ooijen's 3-Step method is disarmingly simple and is the central tenet of the book. The three steps are What, How and What Now, and are translated into Facts, Feelings and Actions. The book works through each of these stages, leading the reader easily from theory, through cases and examples to practice. Towards the end of the book there are two unusual and interesting chapters on supervision and ethical decision-making and on supervision and management and leadership in organisations. Again, the skill of making it easy emerges as van Ooijen uses the 3-Step method to elucidate a model of ethical decision-making and, again, to understand how supervision can be applied both to teams and to organisations.

The blend of theory and practice works well. A down-to-earth style combines with an ability to translate theory into action and practice to help readers understand their own work in systemic ways. van Ooijen moves well beyond the traditional methods of supervision interventions, and outlines innovative and creative ways of implementing supervision: reflective journals are one, but even more powerful is the use of poetry, music and rapid writing.

The book will be an asset for both supervisors and supervisees at all stages of development. Supervisees have, here, a workbook to help them prepare for and engage in supervision that is geared towards their own learning style and learning needs. Supervisors, on the other hand, have a manual for both theory and practice that they can 'dip into' for old and new ways of working as clinical supervisors in a number of settings.

With *Clinical Supervision Made Easy* you get what is stated in the title – a complex subject becomes accessible to supervisors and supervisees at different levels of development.

Michael Carroll PhD,
Visiting Industrial Professor,
University of Bristol

This book presents a step-by-step approach to the art of supervision, presented in an easily read but academically sound framework. The case studies illustrate how the model works and, whilst Els acknowledges theoretical frameworks, the focus is upon practical examples, thus enabling the practitioner to experience the process.

If you are going to buy just one book on supervision, this book should be the one.

Alison J Sullivan CQSW DIP Man,
Freelance Trainer and Life Coach

Clinical Supervision Made Easy is just what is needed within this constantly changing world of health and social care. Els van Ooijen's book provides a structure and an understanding of clinical supervision that is both easy to comprehend and a delight to read. The blend of information and story-telling turns what for some is a very tedious process into an experience that not only stimulates reflective thought but also builds the confidence of both supervisor and supervisee alike.

Maureen Eby, Senior Lecturer,
School of Health and Social Welfare,
The Open University

Acknowledgements

This book could not have been written without my having had the privilege of working with so many good people, both as a supervisor as well as a supervisee. I particularly appreciate the generosity of those people who allowed me to use their work as the basis for some of the examples in the book. Thank you all.

Writing can be a lonely business and other people's interest and willingness to offer constructive criticism is therefore invaluable. So I am especially grateful to all the people who offered helpful comments on the various versions of this work.

My partner, Peter, deserves a special thank you for his patience in putting up with me while I was writing the book and for helping me out with some of the more technical aspects of my computer.

Introduction

FROM TUNNEL VISION TO 'SUPER' VISION

One day in mid-February I popped out to post a letter. It had been dull and overcast for days now so I did not feel inclined to linger outside. As I walked along, however, there was a break in the clouds and a ray of sunshine poured through. Suddenly everything looked different. I noticed the raindrops glistening on tree branches and a few snowdrops in a garden, and felt glad to be outside. The world was the same, yet in an instant, through that ray of sunlight, my view of it had changed completely.

Clinical supervision can be compared to that ray of sunshine in that it can help us to see things differently or more clearly. I could have seen the snowdrops before, but I hadn't. I needed the help of the sun to clarify my vision. Before the sun came out I saw the world through my own thoughts and prejudgements. I thought, 'It is a dull day, there is nothing of interest', so I did not look.

Each one of us sees the world through the window of his thoughts. (Chakravarty 1997:12)

The above experience made me realise that this quote is true, that we do see the world through the 'window' of our thoughts, and so need to keep that window as clean as we can. In clinical supervision we can be helped first to become aware of our thoughts and feelings and then, through reflection, 'clean' them so that we can

1

see what is outside the window. Now, I know that windows have the habit of getting dirty again. I also know that the only thing to do about it is to clean them again, since the cleaner the window, the clearer the view. It shouldn't be surprising that we see the world though the window of our own thoughts, feelings, experience and knowledge – how else would we make sense of it? The important thing is to realise that our view is not the only one, nor is it necessarily superior to anyone else's. As no two people are the same, and we are all shaped by our unique experiences, it is unlikely that any two people will experience the same event in exactly the same way. I have frequently been amazed at the difference between my recollection of an event and those of other people; sometimes it seems that we are not even speaking about the same thing at all.

I have learnt that although each of us probably thinks that we perceive the world 'as it really is' this is not the case. If we did perceive simply 'what is out there' there would not be the amount of conflict and disagreement that there obviously is. 'We see the world not as it is, but as we are … or as we are conditioned to see it' (Covey 1989:228). This is true even for those of us in the helping professions who pride ourselves on our ability to empathise with people. In our interactions, whether with clients or with colleagues, we have a tendency to understand things one way rather than another. Sometimes this means that we feel stuck or that we are missing something, or we may feel less effective than we would like to be without knowing why.

Many of us have occasions when we find it difficult to acknowledge the views of others, particularly if we feel strongly about something. The trouble with such 'tunnel vision' is that it is very limited. It is a wide world out there and we need to keep our vision wide to appreciate it. The 'facts' of any situation have no meaning in themselves, as it is our interpretation of them that gives them meaning. Thus the more we are aware of our habitual ways of seeing things – our prejudgements and our assumptions, in fact our 'map' of our professional world – the more open we will be to the different views of others.

If supervision works well, we are helped to become aware of our 'maps' or the 'lens' through which we see things, so that we develop a 'super' vision. So supervision is not just about unpacking what happens in our interactions; it is also about examining the lens through which we view the interactions themselves.

EXAMPLE: PERSONAL EXPERIENCE CAN ALTER OUR PERCEPTION

Ray, a married man with children, had taken a business degree and now had a reasonable job at a manufacturing company. However, he became increasingly dissatisfied with his working life and wondered whether he had chosen the right career. Then his 2-year-old daughter became very ill and had to be admitted to the local children's hospital. 'I had no idea what nurses did,' he told me. 'It is a very complex job, isn't it? You have to be able to cope with so many different things.' His daughter recovered and Ray decided to retrain as a nurse, which he was able to do as his wife earned a good salary as a computer programmer. 'It will be tough for a few years,' Ray said, 'but I want to do something that has meaning for me. Anyway they told me at the interview that business skills are very much needed in the Health Service, so it's not going to be wasted.'

Ray's example shows how new experiences can radically alter our perception. It also indicates how a changed view can lead to actions so different they could not even have been imagined in advance. I feel that the only way that clinical supervision is going to become an integral part of all helping professions is through people having the actual experience of good supervision, as this can similarly lead to radical changes of view and action that often can't be envisaged beforehand. Adequate training and preparation are therefore essential.

As far as the implementation of clinical supervision in organisations is concerned, I would rather that people started small. I believe that if enough people have positive experiences of supervision that make a difference to the way they practise, a paradigm shift will occur, and powerful change will become possible in the organisation as a whole.

GENERAL BACKGROUND

In the health, social care and voluntary sectors it is increasingly realised that people like to feel valued or they may vote with their feet. Managers in charge of teams and workers dealing directly with clients all need to feel that the jobs they do are recognised as important. In addition, the notion of continuous professional development is now an accepted element of many professions, with re-accreditation contingent on being able to demonstrate this. At an organisational level, staff development should therefore be a priority and not regarded as something people should solely do in their own time and at their own expense. Perhaps paradoxically, those organisations that facilitate their staff's further training and professional development tend to have the lowest levels of staff turnover.

How workers are valued, supported and helped to develop will have a direct impact on the performance of the organisation as a whole. The concept of 'the learning organisation' means that there will be a continuous improvement in the organisation's performance through the continuous professional development of its staff. Supporting individual workers therefore makes sense in organisational terms, as it ensures that the clients, who after all constitute the primary business of the organisation, get a good deal.

PROFESSIONAL DEVELOPMENT THROUGH CLINICAL SUPERVISION

Clinical supervision is increasingly seen as one of the ways in which organisations can demonstrate to their staff that they matter. If an organisation is willing to spend adequate resources on the implementation of clinical supervision, it gives its workers the message that they are important. Indeed, the way in which supervision is implemented in terms of how, when, where and how often it takes place says a great deal about the importance placed upon it by the organisation (Hawkins & Shohet 2000:168). As a worker said recently, 'The fact that my employer thinks that I am important enough to have someone spend time with me on a regular basis to look at how am doing makes me feel valued.'

It seems that supervision, whether clinical, case or managerial, is now a well-known concept in the health, social care and counselling sectors. However, from my meetings with people from a wide range of occupations throughout the country it is becoming increasingly clear that many lack a clear understanding of the nature and purpose of supervision, or the most effective way to practise. Training for supervision is often very short to nonexistent, with the consequence that people often lack a model or framework of what to do and how to do it. It is therefore not surprising that much supervision is not as effective as it could be, which from an organisational point of view is not a good way of investing resources.

Although supervision is much more established in the world of counselling, many counsellors find themselves in the position of having to take the role of supervisor before they have had a chance to undertake any supervision training. In a way, the current situation is an interim stage; although more and more institutions now offer courses in supervision, there are not enough trained supervisors around yet to satisfy the demand.

WHO SHOULD SUPERVISE WHOM?

It can be helpful to receive supervision from someone who is not directly involved with the same clients, patients or users. In my experience, people often opt to receive supervision from someone with a professional 'map' that is similar enough to allow understanding of their work, but different enough not to share the same assumptions or blind spots. Counsellors, for example, may find it helpful to be part of a supervision group that comprises people from different orientations. I have been part of effective, well-functioning groups that included people from psychodynamic, Gestalt, humanistic and cognitive behavioural backgrounds.

Similarly, a nurse working in an accident and emergency department may choose to receive supervision from a nurse in a completely different specialty, such as medicine or psychiatry. I am of course talking here about consultative supervision for experienced professionals. When people are still in training or newly qualified they need to receive supervision from someone from the same professional background or theoretical orientation.

For qualified and experienced professionals, however, clinical supervision is not so much about learning the skills of the job as about looking at their practice through a different lens. Not only will this help them to develop a different and wider perspective, it will also provide them with more choices and flexibility in the way they work.

It seems to me that supervision is increasingly becoming an activity in its own right. This could mean that a trained and experienced supervisor might provide consultative supervision for a number of people from quite different professions, although it may be useful to know a little bit about these professions (Kell 2002). I see such supervisors as using their skills to help supervisees look at their practice in a number of different ways, and thus develop a wider range of options. People often find that having to explain certain elements of their work to a supervisor who is not intimately familiar with all its details can be very helpful in itself. The supervisor's possibly naïve questions, such as 'Tell me, what is your reason for doing that?' can help free up the supervisee's thinking. Perhaps the supervisee had never really given much thought to it as, in her experience, things had always been done in that way. Having to give an explanation might help her to be clearer and perhaps develop a new perspective. I have found, time and again, that being asked such a simple question can help people to stop and think and possibly realise that a particular way of doing things is no longer good or efficient and needs changing.

MULTIPROFESSIONAL PERSPECTIVE

Many people would agree that there is value in a certain amount of shared learning and development across various helping professions. Such shared learning can be an efficient use of resources as it may prevent overlap – different organisations doing the same thing with different people. Also people tend to find a multiprofessional element in training courses really beneficial as it helps them understand other people's working areas and thus promote better links and team-working. Although some training courses in supervision recognise the value of multiprofessional learning, with a few exceptions most books published on the subject of supervision tend to focus on a particular occupational group such as counselling, nursing or social work. Also, up to now there are few books that specifically focus on what to do in a session. The model introduced in this book offers a step-by-step guide on how to practise supervision irrespective of the occupation or professional group.

PERSONAL HISTORY

For many years I wore two hats – the hat of general nursing and the hat of counselling. When I wore my counselling hat, clinical supervision was an integral part of my practice; I do not think I could have functioned effectively without it. Where would I take the stresses and uncertainties, where would I go to be challenged on how I work, if not to supervision? Indeed, the British Association of Counselling and Psychotherapy has long regarded it as unethical for any counsellor to practise without adequate supervision. As far as healthcare is concerned, however, I had never come across any reference to clinical supervision until the early 1990s, when it became increasingly widely debated within nursing as well as in other professions allied to medicine. I found out that hitherto clinical supervision had been practised here and there in mental health nursing and that midwives too had a form of supervision. This greatly excited me. 'At last,' I thought, 'a recognition of the emotional labour involved in healthcare and a realisation that those engaged in any kind of helping profession need to be supported if they are to maintain quality and best practice.'

At the time I was already involved with providing supervision for counsellors, both within an agency and privately, and quickly extended this to nursing and related professions. The experience of providing supervision as well as workshops and courses on the topic for nurses and other health professionals led to the publication of my book *Clinical Supervision: A Practical Guide* in 2000. This focused to a large extent on the preparation needed for supervisees and supervisors alike, as for many healthcare professionals supervision was still a very new concept. The book also included a model, the Double Helix Model of Supervision, which I developed in order to clarify the whole concept of supervision, encompassing an individual as well as an organisational perspective.

I admit that I love doing supervision and have a real passion for it, whether as a supervisor, a supervisee or a trainer. For me, supervision provides the opportunity to really look at what is going on in someone's practice in detail, which can be immensely stimulating both professionally and personally. Of course I am not saying that it is never uncomfortable – all good supervision should challenge us to look at our work honestly so that we can grow and develop. As a supervisee it is wonderful to be able to off-load and be helped to reflect on what is happening. When I wear the hat of the supervisor it is the frisson of not knowing what will be brought that I enjoy (as well as fear, to be honest). Frequently, when someone brings what concerns them to supervision I think, 'Well, I have no idea what's going on and I have even less of a sense what to suggest that may be helpful.' However, over the years I have learnt to, as they say, 'Trust in the process.' Giving it time, attention and consideration, without rushing to find an answer, helping the supervisee to really reflect on what might be going on, is in itself tremendously helpful.

WHY ANOTHER BOOK ON CLINICAL SUPERVISION?

Increasingly it became clear to me that no matter how dedicated and convinced of its usefulness individual practitioners might be, many found the actual practice very difficult. 'Yes, I know all about the reasons for doing clinical supervision and the potential benefits,' an occupational therapist said to me recently. She went on to say, 'I have even managed to get support for it so that we can do it in working hours and a few of us have attended a 3-day workshop to help us to get started.' 'Brilliant,' I said, 'so what's the problem?' 'We get stuck,' she said, 'as we don't always know how to reflect on things in a way that is helpful. Also, in the role of supervisor, I feel such a pressure to come up with the answers. What I would really like is a step-by-step guide on how to actually run a session.' In the past few years I have had quite a few conversations like this, until I thought, 'Why not write a book that does just that?'

Ideally, regular supervision should be a useful habit, something we cannot imagine doing without. Habits consist of three components, desire, knowledge and skills (Covey 1992:42), so all three components need to be in place for supervision to be a positive habit. If one of the three components is missing, clinical supervision may fail. For example, people may have the desire and even some knowledge, but lack the skill. Most literature focuses on knowledge. My aim for this book, however, is to contribute to the development of skill. Desire will hopefully grow as more and more people have positive experiences of supervision.

FOR WHOM HAS THIS BOOK BEEN WRITTEN?

My purpose in writing this book is to clarify and simplify both the structure and process of clinical supervision. It is therefore aimed at those people who have not yet had much experience as a supervisor, although more seasoned supervisors as well as people involved in the training and development of supervisors may also find it useful.

ABOUT THE BOOK

With the permission and cooperation of my supervisees I decided to record my supervision sessions for a while. This enabled me to look at the sessions relatively objectively and get a sense of what it is I actually do. I came to realise that what I actually found myself doing in a session depended on a number of factors. Some of these factors had to do with the supervisees, such as their experience or their openness to challenge or different methods. Other factors appeared to be concerned with our working relationship, or with the nature of the material brought to supervision. I also discovered that all my sessions had a clear framework or map, but that within that framework I used a variety of tools and techniques that I had gleaned from various training courses, books and through experience.

THREE STEPS TO STARTING, DOING AND EVALUATING SUPERVISION

I decided to call my way of working the 3-Step Method. Basically, it comprises three steps: the beginning of a session, the middle and the end. In the book, each of the steps is unpacked to show what needs to happen, and what skills or techniques may be helpful. As the 3-Step method provides a simple structure, and is not based on any particular theory, it can be integrated with other supervision models. I will make clear when I am doing this and why so that you, the reader, can choose whether or not this is appropriate for you. Of course, what I present in this book is my personal integration and readers are therefore encouraged to take from it what seems useful and appropriate and to change or alter what does not. In any case, the way in which I work is by no means set in tablets of stone, and I aim to continue learning and developing and add to the choices available to me. The tools and techniques I present in the book are a result of what I have accumulated over the years. Some methods are my own creation, some I have adapted from others, whereas with others I no longer know where they originally came from. However, wherever possible I will credit the original source.

The examples and case studies in the book are all based on my own experience of practising, teaching and discussing supervision. Where actual bits of transcript are included, permission has been sought and granted from those involved. Other examples are an amalgam of several people and issues, in order to ensure anonymity and confidentiality.

The main focus of the book is the 3-Step method of conducting a supervision session. However, the 3-Step method can also be used as a framework for the setting-up of supervision – whether for individuals or groups, or within an organisation – evaluating supervision, or writing notes of supervision sessions. As far as its use in the actual practice of supervision, the 3-Step method can incorporate other models, theories or approaches. Also, because of its simple structure, it lends itself well to adaptation to different professional contexts.

HOW TO READ THIS BOOK

Although I endorse the importance of gender-neutral language, repeated use of 'he or she' rapidly becomes cumbersome. I therefore alternate my use of 'he' and 'she' for both supervisor and supervisee; the use of one or the other in any particular context has no significance. I have aimed at a conversational, interactive style. In writing the book I wanted to have the sense that I was having a dialogue with you, the reader. I imagined you in the room with me, looking over my shoulder as I wrote. From time to time, therefore, I ask you to stop and think about what you have just read. On other occasions I may present you with a problem and ask you to think about what you would do, because, in my experience, being actively involved like this is helpful in the assimilation, consolidation and remembering of new material.

INTRODUCING THE CHAPTERS

This book is intended to be a practical guide to supervision, which is why I have kept theoretical discussion to a minimum. At the same time, I find that the plethora of models currently available can be confusing, so my aim for Chapter 1 is to provide a simple overview by identifying four different categories of model and then briefly discussing one or two examples of each type. As it is not my intention in this chapter to give an exhaustive account of all the available models, any omissions are by no means intended as a negative reflection.

Supervision will only be effective if the relationship between supervisor and supervisee is good. In Chapter 2, I therefore discuss the importance of getting to know each other first, in order to decide whether both parties feel that they can work together. I introduce the 3-Step method as a simple but comprehensive tool for the development of a working agreement.

Chapters 3–7 are devoted to the actual 'doing' of supervision. In Chapter 3, I outline the 3-Step method of conducting a supervision session and demonstrate its use via a transcript. In the following four chapters I discuss each step in much more detail, including supervision skills, useful techniques and examples from practice. Basically, the three steps refer to the beginning, middle and end of a session. So, in Chapter 4, I discuss Step 1, the 'what' of supervision, which includes helping the supervisee to identify the supervision question, and the clarification of desirable objectives. Two chapters (5 and 6), are devoted to Step 2, the 'how' of supervision, which is the main part of a supervision session. In Chapter 5, I offer a range of techniques to help the reflective process, including creative methods such as artwork and story-telling. Much of what goes on in our interaction with each other happens outside our immediate awareness, so Chapter 6 is devoted to a discussion of unconscious processes in supervision, such as transference, counter-transference and parallel process. Step 3 is the subject of Chapter 7, which comprises a discussion of 'what' to do 'now' after the reflection of Step 2. The five elements of Step 3 are brought together under the acronym LAMEE (Learning, Action, Monitoring, Evaluation and Evidence). In this chapter, I also discuss the importance of adequate 'planning' if a supervision relationship needs to end, for which a 3-Step framework can also be utilised.

The monitoring part of supervision is taken up in Chapter 8, which is devoted to a discussion of ethical decision-making. I suggest a 3-Step framework combined with the 'four principle' approach (Bond 2000) and an ethic of care (Noddings 1986). Group supervision can be very useful, either on its own or in addition to one-to-one supervision. In Chapter 9, I discuss how to use the 3-Step method with groups. Groups offer an opportunity to practise supervision in ways not possible (or more difficult) within individual supervision, so in this chapter I offer a host of tools and techniques designed to make the group sessions as enjoyable and as effective as possible.

Supervision is becoming increasingly important in many organisations within the 'helping sector'. In the last chapter I share some of my thoughts on the relationship between management, leadership and supervision. I also suggest a 3-Step approach to the implementation of the supervision system within an organisation.

I am firmly committed to the importance of lifelong learning, growth and development. For me, that includes feedback on the usefulness of this book. A feedback request is provided at the end of the book, and I will be most interested in any comments you would like to make.

1

Models of supervision

I think it is an illusion to conceive of oneself as working without theories, concepts or methods, because our mind cannot function without them. (Jacoby 1995:83)

Arguably the most important piece of equipment for any supervisor is a conceptual understanding or model of supervision. (Page & Wosket 2001:23)

The usefulness of supervision is increasingly recognised by many of the helping professions, with the effect that there are now quite a few models in existence. In this first chapter I aim to provide some clarity regarding the kinds of models that are available. I do this by first categorising models into four main types, after which I discuss one or more examples of each.

 EXAMPLE: A COMMON PROBLEM

Picture the following. Two people, Peter and Lynn, meet at a conference where mental health policies and strategies are discussed. Peter is an outreach worker at an agency helping people with addiction problems. Lynn works as an occupational therapist within a large healthcare trust. During the coffee break the conversation turns to clinical supervision. 'My supervision is brilliant,' said Peter. 'I could not do the job without it.' 'What is so good about it?' asked Lynn. 'Well,' Peter answered, 'I feel that I can off-load things that are difficult. Not that she tells me what to do, but somehow she manages to help me to find ways of working with people – even when

13

I have been feeling very stuck.' 'That sounds really good, but I don't know how I would do that,' said Lynn. 'I have been told by my manager that I should start supervising a few people, but I feel quite apprehensive. How am I going to do it and what am I supposed to do anyway? I am not sure that I even know exactly what supervision is supposed to be?' 'You might find it helpful to read around the subject,' said Peter. 'I'll give you a few references so you can do some reading and perhaps select a model that is useful for you.'

WHAT ARE MODELS AND WHAT ARE THEY FOR?

A model offers a mental map for ordering complex data and experience. (Proctor 2000:12)

There can be confusion about what is meant by 'models of supervision' as the word 'model' may mean different things to different people. Sometimes the word is used to differentiate between types of implementation, such as managerial versus non-managerial, or individual versus group supervision. Here, the word 'model' refers to a framework or guide for the actual practice of supervision.

To be helpful, models should help us to clarify what is done in supervision, how it is done and why it is done. The function of a model, therefore, is to give us a sense of what we are doing and why we are doing it. In other words, when we practise supervision we need to have a sense of what we are aiming at, so that we know where we should be going. Without such clarity the supervision would be aimless and unlikely to be helpful or effective. Supervision is different from all other aspects of our role as a helping professional. As will be seen in the next few chapters, not only does it require us to use our personal qualities and skills in specific ways, supervision also has its own aims and goals.

TYPES OF MODELS

Regarding the practice of supervision, models can be divided into four main categories:

1. Models of reflection
2. Psychological approach type models

3. Developmental models
4. Supervision specific models.

Let's look at these one at a time.

MODELS OF REFLECTION

Models of reflection comprise a variety of tools and methods that aid the reflective process. They are particularly suited for use by supervisees in preparation for a supervision session. It is a good idea to develop the habit of preparing for supervision by reflecting on our work. Firstly, this will prevent us from becoming dependent on our supervisor and regarding them as a kind of oracle who will always tell us what to do. Secondly, for some issues our own reflection may be sufficient to achieve that 'clearer' vision. Other situations or problems, however, may be more perplexing and it is these that we should be bringing to supervision. I find that making use of reflective models as a pre-reflection can help us make more efficient use of our clinical supervision sessions.

Bond & Holland (1998:107–129) distinguish between logical and intuitive methods of reflection. Intuitive methods include 'top of the head' methods, brainstorming and mind mapping.

Intuitive methods

Top of the head methods involve saying or writing anything that comes to mind regarding a topic, picking out themes afterwards.

Brainstorming is a technique that is often used during workshops or when people come together to work on a specific project. It involves writing down any answers to a specific question that come to mind without censoring anything. It can be useful to do this within a specific time limit. Once the ideas have dried up, Bond & Holland (1998) suggest a rest period, followed by a second, shorter, brainstorming session. The material generated is then sifted for what is useful and what is not.

Mind mapping can be done in stages as follows:

1. Write down the problem, issue or situation in the centre of a large sheet of paper and draw a circle around it.
2. Write down any thoughts that occur around the central circle; draw circles around each thought.
3. Link all circles with a straight line to the central circle.

4. Sit back, look at the map, and add any further thoughts as appropriate, linking them with straight lines. Carry on until no further thoughts occur.

5. Draw two more straight lines from the central circle.

6. Add two 'wild' or 'silly' thoughts.

7. Sit back; does anything else occur to you?

8. This stage is optional but can be useful when people are doing a course or have just read a relevant book: with different colour pens, add further thoughts regarding your course or reading material if they seem relevant. Say how or why and use a different colour for each thought.

9. Now you can rearrange your mind map by deciding which elements seem more important than others, and write them in the form of a main heading with various subheadings.

[Adapted from Bond & Holland (1998:110–111) and Klauser (1986:47–55)]

Logical methods

These include force field analysis and reflective cycles.

A **force field analysis** involves a number of stages as follows:

1. Frozen position: describe the present situation (which is frozen or stuck). You can do this by talking to someone else, by drawing, by 'free fall writing' or by drawing a mind map.

2. Vision: describe how you would like the situation to be – in an ideal world – your 'vision'. Use any method you like, but take care to use feelings as well as facts.

3. Restraining forces: list all the things that get in the way of achieving stage 2.

4. Positive forces: what would push your vision to happen if there were no restraining forces? If this is too difficult or if you cannot think of anything, describe what exists in the present situation that does not make it worse.

5. Look at the four points you have described so far and add anything relevant (from your experience, courses attended, reading that comes to mind).

6. What do you need to do now? What further information do you need? What action might you take?

[Adapted from Bond & Holland 1998:115]

Johns' Reflective Cycle

Johns' Reflective Cycle (Fig. 1.1) is easy to understand and therefore offers a commonsense guide for those new to reflection. The usefulness of the model does, to some extent, depend on the skill and experience of the supervisor as well as on how able and willing the supervisee is to engage with the reflection. It is not meant to be used as a checklist; the questions are suggestions only, starting points, rather than all that need to be asked.

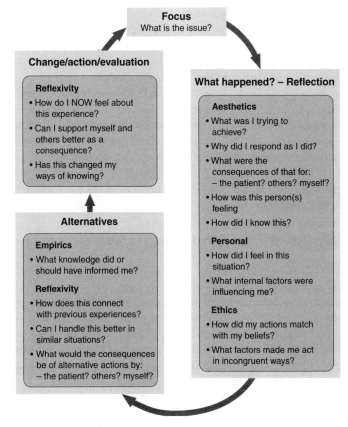

Figure 1.1 Johns' Reflective Cycle (adapted from Johns 1997 in van Ooijen 2000, with permission).

Driscoll's Reflective Cycle

This model comprises three elements:

- What? An event or experience from clinical practice is described, after which some elements are selected for further reflection.
- So what? The event is analysed and any learning from this made conscious.
- Now what? Action is planned and carried out.

Like Johns' model, Driscoll's model (Driscoll 2000:27) offers a straightforward approach to reflection or problem-solving. Its apparent simplicity would make it a useful starting point for those new to reflection or supervision.

The focus of models of reflection is entirely on the supervisee and his or her work. They do not use the supervisory relationship or the process of supervision itself as a vehicle of exploration. People used to working in a more holistic manner may therefore choose a different model, or combine reflective models with a more psychodynamic way of working. Although the models and methods described in this section are useful, I would caution against using them exclusively. Particularly with people new to reflection, there can be a tendency to follow all the steps fairly superficially, thus not achieving as effective a reflection as is desirable. As part of the general toolbox, however, they can provide a supervisor with a rich source of material to be used as and when they are likely to be most helpful.

PSYCHOLOGICAL APPROACH TYPE MODELS

This type of model is most often associated with counselling where supervision originally developed as part of training, which means that, when student counsellors started to practise seeing clients, they would receive supervision for that work as part of their training. In fact, supervised practice is still regarded as an important part of learning how to counsel. There are a number of theories about 'what makes people tick' or 'how best to counsel people'. Some training courses are based on one specific theory, whereas others may take a more eclectic approach, preferring to introduce students to a number of theories. Where students learn about various theories, such integration will be influenced both by the characteristics of the student himself as well as by the area in which he wants to practice. For example a student who is attracted to work in a brief and focused way with people may prefer to learn about cognitive behavioural theories. Others may be interested in working with people over a longer period of several years and may feel that psychodynamic theories have more to offer.

At this point I just want to say that a 'theory' is just a theory. In other words, it represents someone's thoughts rather than the absolute 'truth'. It follows therefore that theories are constantly being revised and updated in light of current scientific knowledge, as well as other people's thinking and experience. For example, Freud first introduced the theory that we have an unconscious mind, after which he developed it further regarding how this mind was developed and what its content and processes might be (its psychodynamic nature). The idea of an 'unconscious mind' has been very influential, although it is by no means the case that everyone subscribes to it. Those who do agree with it, however, do not necessarily still hold on to Freud's explanations of how it works. Freud lived over a hundred years ago, so naturally there are now a great many theories of the unconscious mind and of how knowledge of it can be helpful in our work with clients.

'Same' theory supervision

When people start a training course that adheres to one such theory, for example, it makes sense that the supervision they receive mirrors the theoretical approach of the practitioner. This means therefore that a Gestalt counsellor will supervise using Gestalt methods, a cognitive behavioural counsellor will use cognitive behavioural methods and a psychodynamic-oriented supervisor will use psychodynamic methods, and so on. An advantage of this (approach-specific) type of model is that if you are learning to practise according to a particular theoretical framework, receiving supervision that is congruent with that approach can be very useful, as, in effect, the supervisor acts as a role model for those new to the profession. A possible danger with this kind of supervision is that there is the potential for confusion or blurring of the boundaries between counselling and supervision. A clear contract will therefore need to be set up which clearly sets out those boundaries. (See Chapter 2 for more discussion on the issue of contracting in supervision.)

'Different' theory supervision

As new practitioners gain more and more experience, however, they may choose to have supervision from someone with a different orientation. They do this in the hope that it will provide them with a new way of looking at their work and thus form part of their continuous professional development. Also, many counsellors no longer work according to a discrete theoretical model, instead preferring to form their own integration, which may incorporate a number of theoretical approaches. Experiencing supervision from people with different theoretical backgrounds can greatly facilitate such integration.

DEVELOPMENTAL MODELS OF SUPERVISION

Developmental models are influenced by developmental psychology and focus mainly (but not exclusively) on the development or educative function of supervision. Supervision may be seen as consulting with a 'more seasoned practitioner in the field in order to draw on their wisdom and expertise' (Gilbert & Evans 2000:1). An advantage of this type of model is that it takes account of the supervisee's level of professional development, matching the type of supervision to the knowledge and experience of the supervisee. Although there are quite a few types of developmental model, most incorporate three to five stages of development, starting with the novice worker, through the advanced beginner, via competent worker, very experienced worker to expert (Fig. 1.2) (Hawkins & Shohet 2000:60–65, van Ooijen 2000:6–9).

Although it is clearly sensible to match the way supervision is provided to the developmental stage of the supervisee, problems may occur when such matching does not happen or is incorrect. For example, an experienced worker is likely to become irritated if treated as a beginner; equally, novice workers, irrespective of their profession, are not well served by being expected to function as much more experienced than they are. Neither examples of mismatching are helpful; the latter may even be dangerous. Also, if people's previous educational experiences have been negative, they may approach supervision with trepidation, expecting to be 'shamed' (Gilbert & Evans 2000:13). If such a worker finds herself in a workplace that is shame-based, supervision can be experienced as very destructive.

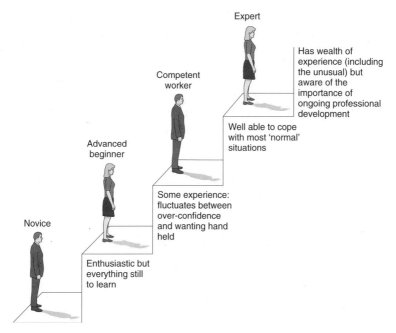

Expert

Has wealth of experience (including the unusual) but aware of the importance of ongoing professional development

Competent worker

Well able to cope with most 'normal' situations

Advanced beginner

Some experience: fluctuates between over-confidence and wanting hand held

Novice

Enthusiastic but everything still to learn

Figure 1.2   Developmental model of supervision.

 THINKING POINT

Have you been in working environments that you experienced as 'shame-based'? What effect did this have on you? What do you think the consequences might be for supervision?

In many helping environments the type of work can be very stressful and the workload high. This can have the effect of everyone working at full stretch, which does not leave much energy for empathising with colleagues who are having problems, or helping those with less experience. People may cope with this type of environment by keeping their head down and 'getting on with the job'. In such an environment it may be hard to ask for help or to admit to finding things difficult as this may be seen as a sign of 'not being up to the job' or of 'making things harder for the others'. Clinical supervision, if implemented sensitively, has much to offer such an environment, but it may take time for practitioners to really trust that they will not be punished for being less than perfect. A developmental approach to supervision can be very helpful as it clarifies the different stages practitioners go through in their professional development. It explains why an 'advanced beginner', for example, can appear fairly competent in one situation and totally out of her depth in another, or why even a competent worker can be 'thrown' by encountering the unusual or unexpected.

As will be discussed in the next chapter, taking the time to get to know each other, before embarking on a supervisory relationship, is crucial for the development of a supportive rather than a destructive working alliance.

SUPERVISION-SPECIFIC MODELS

As supervision has been taken on board by more and more of the helping professions, it has developed increasingly as an activity in its own right. This has lead to an accompanying development of models specifically for supervision. I find it helpful to distinguish them according to their focus as follows:

- Models that focus on the whole concept of supervision
- Models that focus on the tasks and functions of supervision
- Models that focus on the process of supervision
- Models that focus on the structure and process of supervision.

Each type of model approaches clinical supervision from a slightly different angle:

1. Models that focus on the whole concept of supervision: What is clinical supervision about?

2. Models that focus on the tasks and functions of supervision: What is clinical supervision for?

3. Models that focus on the process of supervision: How do we 'do' clinical supervision?

4. Models that focus on the structure and process of supervision: What is clinical supervision for and how do we do it?

Not all supervision models that may be classified in this way have been included in this chapter, as that would fall outside the scope of this book. The models that are discussed have been selected because they are either amongst the most widely used, or because they are judged most versatile and therefore compatible with the 3-Step method, which is this book's main focus. As is clear from the above list, models differ regarding their purpose or aim, so whichever model is chosen will depend on people's type of work and the kind of area in which they practise. In any case, I feel that it is quite legitimate to mix and match and to take various aspects of different models that are considered useful, in order to create a more personal blueprint or guide that works for you.

Models that focus on the whole concept of supervision

This type of model is particularly suited for use on supervision training courses as they help explain and conceptualise all the aspects of supervision, ranging from setting it up at an organisational level, evaluating its effectiveness to what is involved in the actual practice of supervision. Models that focus on the whole concept of supervision are therefore also very useful for those charged with the implementation of a supervision programme in an organisation.

The Double Helix Model of Supervision

The Double Helix Model of Supervision shown in Figure 1.3 (van Ooijen 2000:143) is an example of such a model. Basically, the aim of the model is to give a pictorial view of the following three aspects of supervision:

- Structure: how to set it up.
- Process: how to do it.
- Outcome: how to evaluate it.

Each aspect of supervision is represented by its own double helix, comprising a 'macro' strand and a 'micro' strand. The helices curl upwards together, meet, separate, meet and so on, to reflect the interaction between the individual and the organisation.

The 'macro' strand represents the outside world, the public arena or context within which the supervision takes place. Thus it may denote not only the organisation within which the supervisee works, but also the entire professional environment of professional

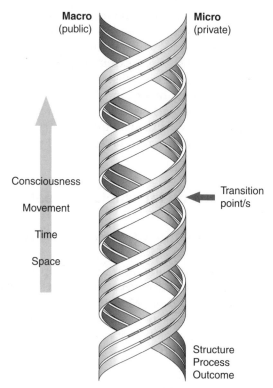

Figure 1.3 The Double Helix Model of Supervision (van Ooijen 2000, with permission).

bodies, registration authorities and so on. Anyone who works for the same organisation is therefore part of that 'macro' strand. However, this does not mean that they all experience that macro world in exactly the same way, as it all depends on people's particular position within it. For example, an individual occupational therapist working within a large mental health institution may experience his professional environment quite differently from a manager in charge of the entire unit. So, depending on the position we take, our perspective may vary considerably.

The 'micro' strand represents the private world of the individual practitioner, which is not immediately accessible to the outside world. Even when two people occupy a very similar position within an organisation, do the same kind of work and perhaps even see some of the same clients, their experience will differ.

This is because no two people are ever the same; we all have our own unique personality and our own personal history, which by definition we do not share with anyone. For example, if five people all attend the same meeting and are asked to give account of what went on, there are likely to be five versions of the event.

 THINKING POINT

Have you experienced this for yourself? What do you think the reasons for it might be?

What happens is that the micro world of the meeting becomes integrated into the micro world of the individual. As we are all different, integration will never be the same; no matter how similar we think we see things to someone else, there will always be differences.

To summarise then, the 'macro' strand of the double helix represents the totality of the environment within which the supervisee works, whereas the 'micro' strand refers to the individual practitioner.

To complement the two helices, four concepts have been added to the model: time, space, movement and consciousness. These join the helices in a continuous upward movement to indicate ongoing growth and development. The helices meet at 'transition points', each of which indicates an insight, an increase in learning, or a greater clarity of vision and consciousness. Integral to the model is the idea of 'cross-over' from the public arena to the private, from macro to micro and vice versa. 'Cross-over' recognises the interdependence of the individual worker and the organisation or context within which they work. People often bring problems to do with organisational dynamics or relations with colleagues to supervision. What the supervisor does is to help them view the issues, both from their own standpoint as well as from the organisational point of view. Being helped to look at the issue from a point of view that is different from their own is often sufficient for the supervisee to know what can be done to solve the problem. Each time a supervisee returns from such a 'cross-over' to the macro strand of the public sphere, he is not quite the same because his vision has altered through the experience.

Models that focus on the tasks and functions of supervision

The Supervisory Alliance Model (Proctor in Cutcliffe et al 2001)

This model originated from the need for supervisory support for practitioners from a wide variety of helping professions, who use counselling skills as part of their work. At the core of the model is the idea that there are three functions of supervision: normative, formative and restorative. Other, more user-friendly, names for the functions are managerial, educative and supportive. Although the entire model is a bit more comprehensive, in practice it is the core that is most widely known and will therefore be used here (Inskipp & Proctor 1993, 1995). The three functions form a 'task framework' that needs to be addressed in supervision.

Knowing what functions should be addressed would be very helpful for Lynn, the occupational therapist mentioned in the vignette earlier in the chapter, as it provides a means of beginning to think what supervision might be for. Although the three functions are usually presented as discrete, I find that in practice there is often an overlap between them. For example, helping a counselling supervisee to reflect on a particular intervention used with a client can be seen as monitoring her practice. It might be useful to check whether the intervention was appropriate, whether it was carried out well, whether the supervisee was qualified and experienced enough to carry it out safely or whether it was actually effective. However, it is also supportive to be able to talk about what was done and to consider what worked well and what was not particularly successful. As result of the reflection, the counsellor may have gained a better insight into the client's problems. She may have learnt what kind of interventions work well with this client, which are less helpful and what the reasons for this might be. All this is part of the formative function. Lastly, the fulfilment of the three functions is not just the responsibility of the supervisor. It goes without saying that the process is two-way; there are two people involved, therefore both have to share the responsibility, although views differ regarding the extent to which this responsibility is shared. The Supervisory Alliance Model can easily be integrated with a developmental approach to supervision. In this case there may be a greater emphasis on the formative or educational function if the supervisee is still in training or only recently qualified.

Table 1.1   Functions and tasks of supervision

Function	Tasks
Restorative/supportive	To counsel To consult
Formative/educative	To set up a learning relationship To teach
Normative/managerial	To monitor administrative aspects To monitor professional ethical issues To evaluate

The Seven Tasks Model

Carroll developed this model as a result of his research into how counsellors see supervision (Carroll 1996). The seven tasks that he identified are:

1. To monitor administrative aspects
2. To set up a learning relationship
3. To teach
4. To evaluate
5. To monitor professional ethical issues
6. To counsel
7. To consult.

What strikes me about the Seven Tasks Model is that the tasks appear to be congruent with the three functions of the Supervisory Alliance Model. I find it helpful to group them as shown in Table 1.1. Both models are useful in that they provide a clear map of what supervision is for. In other words, they clarify its purpose and outline some of the ways in which this can be achieved.

Models that focus on the process of supervision

The Double Matrix or Seven-Eyed Model
(Hawkins & Shohet 2000)

This model, which was developed for use across all helping professions, does not attempt to structure a session or series of sessions. Instead it comprises two large circles, which are called matrices: the Therapy Matrix and the Supervision Matrix (see Fig. 1.4). Each matrix is further divided into three smaller circles, so-called 'modes'

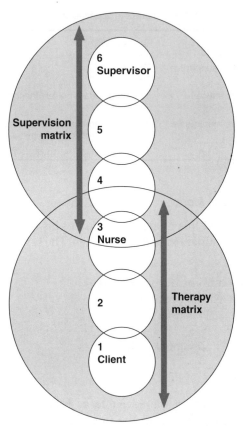

Figure 1.4   The Double Matrix Model (adapted from Hawkins & Shohet 1989 in van Ooijen 2000, with permission).

of supervision. Within the therapy matrix the focus is directly on what happens between the worker and the client; within the supervision matrix the focus is on how the worker–client relationship is reflected in what is going on between supervisor and supervisee.

According to Hawkins and Shohet, supervisors tend to lean to one of two distinct styles of supervision: those who function mainly within the therapy matrix and those who work mainly within the supervision matrix. Supervisors who work mainly through getting supervisees to reflect on their practice (using a model of reflection) would fall in the therapy matrix where the focus is on 'what happened out there'. In the supervision matrix, attention is paid to 'what is happening here', in the interaction between

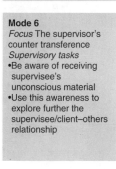

Mode 1
Focus The client/situation
Supervisory tasks
Ask supervisee to:
•Describe client/situation
 in detail
•Challenge assumptions
•Watch for 'filter' through
 which information is seen
 and reported

Mode 2
Focus The what, why,
how of the supervisee's
actions/interventions
Supervisory tasks
Help supervisee to:
•Become aware of
 stuck thinking
•Generate new options

Mode 3
Focus The system
(supervisee and
client/others)
Supervisory tasks
Help supervisee to:
•'Stand outside' the
 situation and see the
 'pattern and dynamic of
 the relationship'
•Bring client's
 transference to
 supervisee's awareness

Mode 4
Focus The supervisee's
counter transference
Supervisory tasks
Help supervisee to:
•Bring their counter-
 transference to aware-
 ness
•Explore all forms of
 counter transference,
 creating 'space to
 respond rather than
 react'

Mode 5
Focus The supervisory
relationship
Supervisory tasks
•Identifying parallel
 processes

Mode 6
Focus The supervisor's
counter transference
Supervisory tasks
•Be aware of receiving
 supervisee's
 unconscious material
•Use this awareness to
 explore further the
 supervisee/client–others
 relationship

Figure 1.5   The six modes of supervision and their main focus.

supervisor and worker and what light this might shed on 'what happened out there', between worker and client. In the second edition of their book, Hawkins and Shohet added a seventh mode or eye, which represents the wider organisational context in which both the supervisee's work and the supervision itself takes place. As the Double Matrix Model is mainly concerned with the process of supervision, it is compatible with the 3-Step method, which is the focus for the remainder of this book. (Step 2 concerns the process of supervision.) I will therefore explain the main focus of each mode a little further, as well as the relevant tasks of the supervisor (see Fig. 1.5).

Models that focus on structure and process

The Cyclical Model

This model incorporates the main concepts of contracting, focus, space, bridge and review (Fig. 1.6), and was developed for use in counselling supervision. Each concept contains a further five or

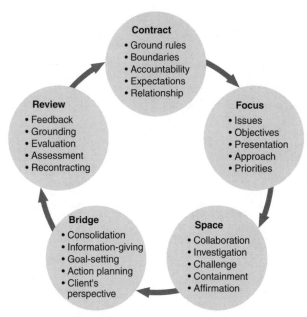

Figure 1.6   The Cyclical Model (adapted from Page & Wosket 1994 in van Ooijen 2000, with permission).

six elements, all of which have to be addressed for the supervision to be effective.

As is clear from the name, in this model the supervision process is seen as cyclical. For example, the discussion taking place in the review section may well lead to the need for recontracting and so on. Deciding on the focus for the session is the next task. This involves what is brought for discussion and how it is introduced, as well as ascertaining the supervisee's objective in doing so. If there is more than one issue, a decision needs to be made regarding which is more important, or which is going to be discussed first. In the 'space' section, the actual reflection on practice takes place, followed by the 'bridge' section. Here links are made between what was discussed in the session and how the worker is going to take it back to their actual practice.

A slight disadvantage of the model is that for some people the subdivisions of each of the five elements make it seem a bit intimidating. However, I find the Cyclical Model particularly useful for those new to supervision as it is comprehensive and can provide a basis for teaching people how to supervise. Each of the five concepts can in fact provide a basis for a teaching session. For example, if they want to, people can practise contracting over and over, until they feel they have achieved a sense of mastery without being concerned about moving around the cycle. Having mastered the concept of contracting they can move onto focusing and so on.

The model may also be used in group supervision, where it can provide a structure for the running of the group. It is, for instance, always a good idea to start a supervision session with a reminder of the contract. For example, the group facilitator may ask: How much time do we have? How shall we allocate it? She may also like to remind people of any other boundaries or ground rules that have been agreed.

CONCLUSION

In this chapter I have explained how models of supervision might be categorised into four main types. One or more examples of each type were discussed briefly, as well as some of their advantages and disadvantages. In the next few chapters I will introduce the 3-Step method to conducting a supervision session, which can be used in conjunction with some of the models discussed.

Questions for reflection

- Have you been using a model of supervision? If so, how would you categorise it?

- If you have not been using a model, which type do you feel most drawn to at this stage, either as a supervisee or as a supervisor?

- What are your reasons for this choice?

2

Three steps to starting supervision

The relationship is an area in supervision that requires clear contracting and negotiation. (Carroll 1996:55)

Relationship is the dynamic element of supervision. (Holloway 1995:41)

In this chapter I first discuss helpful skills, qualities and attitudes, both for supervisors and for supervisees. Next I set out how the 3-Step method may be used to get to know each other and to develop a working agreement.

 EXAMPLE: THE IMPORTANCE OF DOING SOME 'GROUNDWORK'

Liz came to see me in a bit of a state. 'I'm fed up,' she said. 'I know he's my supervisor and everything, but that doesn't give him the right to talk to me the way he does.' I pushed a mug of tea across the kitchen table and prepared to listen. Liz is an experienced nurse, who, over the years had done a fair bit of personal and professional development. As part of a course in counselling skills she was currently on a placement with a voluntary organisation that provides services for young people with a variety of problems, including mental health issues. Liz had felt that the placement would suit her down to the ground, as it would help her to combine her existing nursing experience with her developing counselling skills. 'You were really looking forward to your placement, weren't you,' I said. 'Yes,' answered Liz, 'and I was particularly pleased to be supervised by Ian, as he's got such a good name and has so much experience.'

So what was the problem? It transpired that, like many organisations in the voluntary sector, the services provided by the agency were in high demand, which meant that everybody was working flat out. Ian's workload was such that he only had time to see his supervisees at the allotted times and therefore tended to get straight down to business. 'I don't think he realises how experienced I am,' said Liz. 'Judging from the way he talks to me he assumes that I've never done anything in my entire life.' 'Why not talk with him about that?' I said. 'How else is he going to know?' 'Yes, I know,' said Liz. 'In fact I've made a special appointment to see him. I just wanted to let off steam first as I don't want to blow it. Sorry about that.' 'You're welcome,' I said. 'What are friends for? Next time it's my turn though.' We both laughed.

What Liz's example indicates is that it is important to do some groundwork first before starting to engage in the process of supervision.

ESSENTIAL PREREQUISITES FOR EFFECTIVE SUPERVISION

SKILLS, QUALITIES AND ATTITUDES

Although it is claimed that supervision has been around since the time of Freud, it is only in the last few decades that it has begun to be taken seriously in the fields of health, social care and counselling. When I first became a supervisor I had not received any formal training or preparation to do so. At the time this was not unusual. It was assumed that, if you were a competent and experienced professional, then you would naturally be able to supervise others. For my part I realised fairly soon that I did not have a clear idea what to do, so I modelled myself on the supervision I had received myself. Although this helped a bit, it did not prevent me from feeling out of my depth on quite a few occasions. This was not helped by my realisation that my own supervisors had not really received any preparation for the activity either. How could I be sure that I was doing the right thing in copying them? Luckily it was not long before I was able to take advantage of some training courses and workshops. This was immensely helpful. Not only did the training give me confidence, it also made me realise that, with some refocusing, I could use many of my existing skills and qualities.

So what are the skills, qualities and attitudes needed for supervision? The best supervisors are those who can make really good use of their own supervision. In other words, they know what it is like to be a supervisee and therefore do not find it difficult to have a sense of what a session might feel like for their own supervisees. I believe that the extent to which supervisors are able to help their supervisees reflect is intimately related to the level of reflection they are capable of for themselves.

KNOWING WHAT WE WANT

I don't know about you, but I tend to go blank when someone asks me 'What do you want?' It can be really difficult to know straightaway what that is. Somehow this seems to apply particularly to birthday or Christmas presents, as the things I really want (a Greek island, a 4-day weekend every week, my books becoming bestsellers so that I can retire) are invariably outside people's capacity to provide.

As far as supervision is concerned, though, it is a good idea for the other person to know what it is you would like them to provide. This is useful even if they disagree with it, because, as will be seen in the second part of this chapter, it can then form the basis for a frank discussion.

 THINKING POINT

Take a break from reading and think about the following two questions:

1. As a supervisee what skills and qualities would you like your supervisor to have?
2. As a supervisor what skills and qualities would you like to see in the people you supervise?

For the first question it may be helpful to think of all the people you have come across in your life who have helped you in some way or another. Perhaps there was a teacher who pointed you in the right direction when you had an essay to write, or a career officer who helped you to clarify your choice of work or study? Or maybe there was someone who helped you when you first started work when you felt that you were doing everything wrong. What did they do and what qualities do you associate with them? You may also like to think of yourself as you are now. What would help you in your current position, what is it you feel you need? How would you like to be helped not only to maintain the quality of your work, but also to help you move on and develop further?

For the second question imagine yourself working with the perfect supervisee. Or, if you are already supervising, think of those people that you enjoy working with.

Take your time and write down everything that occurs to you, even the silly wishes that you would not like to share with anyone else. They are still useful for you to know about and perhaps bear in mind when you meet the other person.

When I ask the above two questions at workshops, I am often impressed with just how much people can come up with. Although there is often a great deal of similarity between what people want, there are nearly always some surprises. I think this is good as it is a reminder that we are all different and that we can never assume that we know what it is that people want and need.

Table 2.1 sets out a range of skills, qualities and attitudes. As you will notice, there are quite a few that are useful for both the supervisor and the supervisee, although the way in which they are used may be different. Sometimes people think that supervision is something that we receive or that is done to us. By implication that means that the supervisor is the one who is doing all the work. Nothing could be further from the truth. Successful supervision demands the active involvement of both parties and the willingness to do so is therefore a first requirement.

Giving honest mutual feedback is also very important. As the example at the beginning of the chapter showed, it was no good for Liz to complain to a third person that her supervisor was not helping her. The person to take this sort of thing up with is your supervisor. If you are unable to sort things out between you, a way needs to be found to end the relationship so that both of you have a chance to work with someone else. This need not be seen as a failure. It is a fact of life that we do not get on with everybody and that

Table 2.1 Desirable skills, qualities and attitudes

Both supervisor and supervisee	The supervisor	The supervisee
Willingness to be actively involved	Keeping appropriate boundaries	Listening skills
Communication skills	Active listening (reflect, paraphrase, summarise)	Accept support
Commitment	Questioning	Accept praise
Motivated	Empathise	Accept constructive criticism
Openness	Support	Accept responsibility for own practice
Non-defensiveness	Supportive challenge	Describe issues clearly
Relationship-building	Confrontation	Prioritise
Approachable	Facilitation	Clarify
Honesty	Validation and affirmation	Analyse
Trust	Creating a safe space	Reflect
Courage	Emotional literacy	
Generosity	Cope with difficult emotions	
Evaluating own process honestly	Able to face the negative (in self and others)	
Awareness of strengths and weaknesses – and willingness to learn more about them	Appropriate self-disclosure	
	Ability to tolerate 'not knowing'	
Focus on own thoughts, feelings and emotions, attitudes and values	Ability to create and stay with the 'space'	
Aware of own safety	Resisting temptation to work too hard	
Self-reflection	Internal supervision skills	
Linking reflection to action	Reframing	
Generating ideas for action	Empowerment	
Decision-making	Facilitate people's growth and development	
Giving and receiving constructive feedback	Personal and professional authority	
Accept responsibility	Leadership	
Ability to learn from mistakes	Giving feedback appropriate to the supervisee's level of experience	
Sense of humour (it helps, honest)		

we work better with some people than with others. There has to be enough of a match for it to work. It is great if both parties have a genuine sense of curiosity and adventure about supervision, so that it is not seen as 'yet another thing we have to do' but as something that will help us grow and develop.

This may seem an enormous list, no let me rephrase that: it is an enormous list. But look at it honestly, and you will find that you already have many of the qualities mentioned. Also, I hope no-one is expecting either themselves or the other person to be totally competent in each and every one of the items on the list. That would be very frightening. Rather, I see the list (which is not meant to be exhaustive, by the way) as a useful reminder of what is desirable and what it is useful to aim for. For further reading on how we can prepare ourselves for the roles of supervisor or supervisee see van Ooijen (2000:57–101). Also, in Chapters 4–6, supervisory skills and qualities are discussed in more detail, as well as how they relate to the tasks of supervision in terms of the 3-Step method.

DEVELOPING A WORKING AGREEMENT

The relationship between supervisor and supervisee is the most important aspect of supervision. No matter how experienced the supervisor and how potentially willing the supervisee, if the relationship is not good the supervision is unlikely to be as effective as it might be. In a way it is the relationship between supervisor and supervisee that holds the process of supervision. It is therefore important to take the time to get to know each other and to listen to our own feelings about the other person (Page & Wosket 2001: 95–96). Taking the time to get to know each other will help develop trust and safety, both of which are essential, as in their absence the supervisee will not bring sensitive material and the supervision will not be as effective as it could be. I prefer a relational, humanistic, co-worker relationship to a hierarchical one. In other words, a relationship that respects the supervisee, and one that does not infantilise or shame. A co-worker stance does not mean an abdication of authority. Rather it indicates a personal authority. Power with, rather than power over, the supervisee. Without personal authority, which is based on your own knowledge (including self-knowledge) and experience, a supervisor is unlikely to be effective. In other words, supervisees need to feel that their supervisors know what they are talking about. So in the relationship, which is an alliance between supervisor and supervisee, such authority needs to be earned and deserved in the eyes of the supervisee.

I prefer the term 'working agreement' to 'contract' as I feel it describes more accurately what actually happens when we start to work with someone. Basically the supervisor and supervisee agree to work with each other for a while, but are free to change the way in which it is done by mutual agreement. The three steps form a useful way to set about developing such an agreement as it helps both parties to consider important questions that need to be addressed.

STEP 1: THE 'WHAT' OF A WORKING AGREEMENT

Questions to address

Questions to address regarding the relationship:

- What is our relationship and what are our feelings about working together?

Questions to address regarding each other may include:

- What is your professional role?
- What kind of a person are you?
- What is the purpose of supervision?
- What are you looking for?
- What is your experience of supervision?
- What do you think of me?

What is our relationship and what are our feelings about working together?

These are crucial first questions to consider as they set the scene for all other aspects of the relationship. Therefore, whether I talk with a new supervisor for my own work or whether I meet with a potential new supervisee the first thing we need to talk about is how we came together. As part of our initial 'getting to know each other' chat, I may ask if they have had supervision before:

- Tell me, what prompted you to seek supervision now? Or
- What prompted you to look for a different supervisor?

I would go on to ask:

- What are you hoping for if we start to work together?
- What would you definitely *not* want and why?

Of course this 'getting to know each other' stage goes both ways and the supervisee may therefore like to reciprocate. The supervisor could help by asking questions such as:

- What would you like me to tell you?
- What would be useful for you to know about me?

What needs to be put on the table is any pre-existing relationship such as colleague, manager/staff, friend or acquaintance, friend of a friend, teacher/student and so on. Both of you need to be clear about this relationship and how you both feel about now negotiating a different way of being together.

Even if you have never met before, whether or not you have a choice in working together is bound to influence things. If both supervisor and supervisee work for the same organisation they may have little choice in the matter, which may on occasion be a source of resentment on either or both parts. You as the supervisor may feel that you already have enough to do without being given even more work, whereas your potential supervisee might have hoped for a different person. I feel that it is best to have this out in the open right from the beginning. If this is not done any resentment or disappointment can really get in the way of working together. If, on the other hand, you can both be honest about how you feel, you can discuss how you are going to work with it and you may well find that the resentment disappears.

What is your professional role?

If you are both from the same professional group you will already have a great deal of understanding about each other's work. However, I feel that it is still important to talk more about this, as we can never take for granted that we always see things the same way. It is therefore worth checking out how each of you views your profession and your own role within it.

A hospital social worker, who mainly works with elderly people, told me that he finds it important to have an understanding of how particular diseases, such as a stroke or heart condition, can affect them. To him this seemed common sense. However, it was not a view shared by some of his colleagues, who felt that this was stepping outside his professional boundaries. Counsellors may have different points of view too in that they may not share the same theoretical orientation. However, even if they do, their particular 'take' on, say, the person-centred approach or a Gestalt way of working may vary. It is good to talk about all this as part of getting to know each other, both as professionals and as people.

Many people are asked to supervise someone within their own work area, as it can be very useful to have a good understanding of the supervisee's work. However, a potential danger with having supervision from someone whose work context is the same is that the supervisor may find it more difficult to be objective and may even share the same blind spots (Bramley 1996:30). An added complication arises if the role of clinical supervisor is combined with that of manager, as in that case you need to balance a number of roles, which may on occasion be in conflict (van Ooijen 2000:26–27). Care needs to be taken that the monitoring function of supervision is balanced by the functions of support and facilitating the supervisee's development. From my discussions with various professional groups I find that the demands of the job can be such that the monitoring function often takes centre stage at the expense of the other two functions.

If you are asked to supervise someone from a different professional group it is important that you have an understanding of that person's work. Sometimes people find it easier to supervise someone whose job is very different to theirs as that means that they really have to ask a lot of questions in order to get a sense of it. People who already have some knowledge, on the other hand, such as a nurse and an occupational therapist, may feel that they already have an idea of the other person's job, which may prevent them from listening as well as they might and perhaps make premature judgements.

What kind of a person are you?

People differ to the extent that they like to know the other person. Some supervisors really only want to know the minimum details about a person's life, whereas others prefer to get a sense of the other as an individual apart from their professional role. However, even if we never talk about anything other than our work, the way in which we do this will reflect how we are as people. We all form an impression of people the minute we set eyes on them. I am amazed at how often my first impression is quite different from the one I have once I get to know people. I think that in a way our first impressions say more about us than about the other person as we compare the person we see with other people we know (or have known in the past) who shared some of the same characteristics. We do this so quickly that often we are not even aware that it is happening. Our society is full of ideas, stereotypes and prejudices about people, which can really get in the way of getting to know someone (van Ooijen & Charnock 1994:60–65, 95–99). Since the supervisory relationship is key to the effectiveness of the supervision, it is important to check out whether there are any such obstacles to its development.

What is the purpose of supervision?

This is a big issue and one we really need to spend time on, as agreement regarding the purpose and process of supervision is crucial. Most people in the helping professions agree with the three functions of supervision as discussed in Chapter 1 (Proctor in Cutcliffe et al 2001). Yet how these three functions are understood can vary a great deal.

What is the appropriate balance between support and challenge?

I have heard people say that their supervisor is too supportive and that they therefore were not always sure whether they could believe them. To me that is a misunderstanding of what it means to be supportive. If I had a supervisor who thought that everything I do or say is wonderful and never questioned or challenged anything, I do not think that I would feel supported at all. To the contrary, I would feel that he was not interested or not experienced enough to help me gain a fresh perspective. For me, to be supported means to be listened to attentively. It means that the other person really wants to know and understand what is going on and therefore will need to ask (often searching) questions.

To be supportive also means caring sufficiently about the other person to challenge them and disagree with them. It is because I know that my supervisor will challenge me when he sees something I have not seen, or views it differently, that I can take his praise seriously. In other words, support without challenge may be perceived as unsupportive. Conversely, challenge without support can be destructive. Support and challenge go hand in hand. Support helps us take on board challenge, and the presence of challenge helps us to believe the support. This may sound simple, but the ability to provide the right balance of support and challenge is a special supervisory skill. What makes matters even more complex is that supervisees differ regarding the balance they need. Some prefer high support with some challenge, some like it to be fifty–fifty, whereas others thrive on a diet of high challenge. All this is part of getting to know each other and needs to be discussed before starting to work together.

Does the purpose of supervision include counselling?

It is of particular importance that the supervisor never elicits any information about the supervisee's personal life. (Fordham in Kugler 1995:45–46)

When I first started to supervise people the British Association of Counselling and Psychotherapy had not yet stipulated that counselling and supervision should not be mixed; indeed, at the time, there was not much supervision training available. A person came to see me who wanted me to function both as counsellor and as supervisor. I was not sure how this would work, but agreed to give it a try. At the beginning of a session the person would say what was wanted so that I knew which mode to go in and where the focus should be. So, although this seemed clear in theory, in practice I, as the counsellor and supervisor, found it difficult and confusing. I felt uncomfortable with the mixing, it just did not feel right to engage in deep personal exploration when in the previous session we had been talking as colleagues. I explained my difficulty to the supervisee/client and said that a choice had to be made. I was happy to continue either as counsellor or as supervisor, but not as both.

I now regard the experience as a useful one to have had. Without it I might be less clear on the reasons for the separation. It also clarified for me how very different the two activities are. Although both counselling and supervision involve a relationship between people, the nature of the relationship is very different. Any relationship needs time to grow and develop; above all the people concerned need to get used to each other and feel safe. I found that mixing the two types of relationship made this much more difficult. For me it was confusing and uncomfortable, and potentially unsafe. Therefore, if a supervisee, for whatever reason, strays into unwarranted self-disclosure and I feel the pull to stray into counselling,

I see it as my responsibility as a supervisor to prevent this from happening. I find it easiest to say something like 'I can see that this is a difficult issue for you, but it would be inappropriate for us to work on it further as we would be crossing the boundaries of supervision.' I may remind them of our working agreement and will also check whether they have somewhere else where they can take it. If the issue of boundaries has been clearly discussed in the working agreement this is never a problem. In fact, supervisees tend to be pleased to be reminded of the boundary. As one person said, 'Even though I felt I wanted help with this issue, if you had fallen for it I feel sure that I would have resented it later. In fact, I might well have stopped coming to you for supervision.'

Sometimes the supportive function of supervision can lead to confusion regarding the difference with counselling. This is not surprising, as there are certain similarities. A set time is set aside on a regular basis for one person to talk to another. This other person listens attentively and employs a range of skills, some of which are the same as in counselling. However, using some of the same skills does not mean that the actual activity is the same. For example, we may be good at catching a ball; that is a particular skill we have. There is, however, a world of difference between being the official ball catcher in a game of professional cricket or throwing a ball around with a few toddlers. This is because the context and the purpose are different. Both cricket and playing with toddlers require the skills of being to catch a ball, but that is where the similarity ends, as each activity demands a range of completely different skills. It would be inappropriate to start treating the rest of the team as if they were a group of toddlers; similarly the toddlers would be left rather bewildered if they were treated and expected to behave like a professional cricket team.

A similar distinction applies to the difference between counselling and supervision. Although supervision can be therapeutic it is not counselling or therapy as it differs in focus and purpose. Confusion can arise sometimes because of certain similarities between counselling and supervision, such as regular, time-boundaried meetings, attention to one person (the supervisee), the importance of the relationship, confidentiality and safety. Some of the skills may seem similar, particularly the skills of active listening such as reflection, paraphrasing and summarising. But there is an important difference: in counselling the focus is on the client herself, her inner world and on how past experiences may affect how she perceives and reacts to people and situations in the present. So counselling is about the development of greater personal awareness of one's inner landscape. In supervision, the focus is not on the inner world of the supervisee, but on their work. Sometimes it can happen, particularly if a supervisee is feeling fragile or upset about something, that they may appear to want to talk about some personal issues. I believe it to be a mistake to fall in with it because, as the above example shows, it will muddy the waters and lead to confusion. However, the context and purpose in which they are used are very different.

Of course it is true that as helping professionals we do use ourselves in our work, but that does not mean that we should use our supervision to work on a personal problem. It can happen that during a supervision session it transpires that there is a personal problem underlying some problem with the work. Clearly, it would not be very helpful to ignore it; on the other hand, it would be inappropriate for the supervisor to then switch into counselling mode. What is helpful though is to discuss with the supervisee how and where she could go for help.

How are the educative and normative functions to be addressed?

How the other two functions (educative and normative) are seen also needs to be addressed. For example, some supervisors may regard the educative function as meaning that they will engage in a certain amount of direct teaching. This may be appropriate if the supervisee is a trainee or has chosen the supervisor in order to learn about a different way of working. Even in those cases, though, I feel that it is important for the supervisor to always first ascertain the supervisee's knowledge, experience and ideas. It can be very annoying to have to listen to a lecture on something you already know, or not to be given the opportunity to develop the answer yourself, helped by some gentle prompts.

It is therefore important that the supervisor has a sense of the level of experience of the supervisee so that the supervision can be matched to the supervisee's developmental level. Such development does not just involve the supervisee's professional development. The supervisor also needs to be sensitive to the supervisee's level of personal development and self-awareness (van Ooijen 2000:58–64). This is because we can only really make use of what we are ready to receive. For example, it is no good engaging a teacher to teach our 6-year-old A level mathematics. No matter how brilliant the teacher, our child will not be ready to receive this information. An ancient saying states: 'When the student is ready the teacher will appear.' Perhaps the same is true of supervisors.

The normative or managerial function can be seen in different ways. What both parties mean by this function needs to be clear. I like to think of this function as the practitioner monitoring her own practice, but helped in this by the supervisor. If your supervisor is also your manager there are of course additional issues. In any case, even if both of you are quite happy at being asked to work together you need to discuss how any pre-existing relationship can be kept separate from the supervision relationship. What would not be helpful is if the manager/supervisor were to stop the supervisee on the stairs in order to receive an update on how things are going with a particular client. Of course, being stopped on the stairs for this kind of conversation is never a good idea; however, it would be disastrous if material from clinical supervision sessions were to spill over in this way. Apart from the possibility of being overheard and confidentiality therefore being compromised, it will probably lead to the supervisee feeling unsafe and the supervision itself becoming less effective. If, however, you can agree to really keep what is discussed within the supervision sessions, as well as the way in which it is discussed, distinct from your everyday relationship, the supervision is much more likely to be effective and successful.

What are you looking for?

This question follows on naturally from the above discussion on the purpose of supervision. Being clear on what it is the supervisee wants and needs from supervision can do much to prevent any problems later on. As Liz's example at the beginning of this chapter shows, a failure to do so can lead to much frustration and crossed purposes. This kind of question also helps the supervisee to be clear on what it is they actually want. The kinds of answers people may give vary, but may include:

- I want a space where I can say what is important about my work.
- I want somewhere where there is holding of difficult things.
- I want somewhere where I can be upset and say what I can't say elsewhere.

- I want a place where I am challenged.
- I want someone to help me become aware of my blind spots.
- I want help in monitoring my practice.
- I want help in being opened up so that I can become more creative.
- I want to be seen both as the person I am and for the work that I do.
- I want to be validated for the work that I do.
- I want help in continuing to remain curious and to grow, develop and learn.

I have noticed that people's answers to the question can usually be categorised somewhere within the three functions of supervision (supportive, normative, educative). It can also be useful to ask:

- What is it you really want, but find difficult to ask? Or
- What is it you really do not want from supervision?

This will help the supervisee to reflect on and express what may be difficult and will help to begin to create the safety that is needed. As a supervisor I like to keep a space open for any requests or wishes that may be difficult to voice, or which the supervisee may not be consciously aware of (Bramley 1996:33).

What is your experience of supervision?

It is good to encourage people to talk about their previous experience of supervision as to some extent it is all we can go by; how else can we make sense of the world? I'm sure that experiences of supervision are as varied as the people involved. We cannot therefore assume that we know what someone is going to be like just because they are a supervisor or supervisee. Our experiences may be positive, negative or indifferent.

We also may like to have an idea of the other person's experience. As a supervisor I like to know whether a new supervisee has had experience of supervision and what that was like, as it can affect how we work together. I may ask questions to find out what it was like, what worked, what did not work, what was difficult and what would they like to be different with me. All this will help to give me an indication of how the supervisee may need me to be. It may be useful to come back to these questions from time to time as processes and situations often need to be repeated several times before we have learnt what there is to learn.

I also like to encourage a potential supervisee to enquire about my experience as that will help them to decide whether or not I am the right person for them.

What do you think of me?

This is a question we will probably not ask but which is likely to be in our minds all the same. We all want to be thought well of and are unlikely to feel comfortable if we think that the other person does not like us or has a low opinion of us. I do not think it is reasonable to expect to be able to work with everyone – we are only human after all.[1]

STEP 2: THE 'HOW' OF A WORKING AGREEMENT

Questions to address

- How are we going to take this forward?
- How are we going to work together?
- How will we ensure safety and confidentiality?
- How do we see accountability?
- How will we resolve any problems between us?
- How will we know whether we are effective and working well?
- How long do we want to agree to work together?

How are we going to take this forward?

Having asked each other the kind of questions discussed under Step 1, we are now in a position to decide whether or not we feel we can work together. We may feel that we both need to think about it before committing ourselves. In this case we may decide to contact each other again in, say, a week. If, on the other hand, we feel we would like to work together, we may like to agree to meet again soon. This would give us a chance to think about what exactly it is we want and perhaps to ask further questions that did not occur to us previously. However, it is also possible that Step 1 was very

[1]For further reading on the supervisory relationship, see van Ooijen (2000:25–55).

straightforward and that both parties are keen to get on with Step 2; in which case, why not?

Sometimes other people need to be involved at this stage. If a supervisee is in training, for example, she may need to ask for the supervisor to be approved by the training organisation. Or perhaps the supervisee's manager needs to be involved in deciding whether the supervisor is appropriate.

How are we going to work together?

This involves the nitty gritty of the supervision process. First of all the practicalities need to be discussed, such as: How often will we meet and where? How long will the sessions be? How will holidays and cancellations be handled? (van Ooijen 2000:42–43). I learnt the importance of this the hard way when someone I had agreed to start supervising kept altering the date for the first supervision appointment without giving me sufficient notice. This caused me a good deal of inconvenience and also made me feel resentful and devalued – all this before we had even started working together! Now I insist on a minimum cancellation period of 48 hours. Not only will this help me to use the cancelled time more productively, it also gives the message that the supervision has to be taken seriously.

Next you need to talk about the structure and process of the actual supervision sessions. People vary in what they find helpful. Some supervisors are happy to leave what is brought to supervision entirely up to the supervisee, whereas others like to take a more active part. There is something to be said for a supervisor having a good overview of all aspects of a supervisee's work. I find that, even if an issue is not directly related to working with a client, it may still be useful to talk about it in supervision. If we are engaged in a helping type of job, everything we do will eventually, directly or indirectly, have an impact on the clients. This, in itself makes every aspect of the work legitimate supervision material. On the other hand, I would certainly challenge a supervisee who never brought any client material, despite having regular contacts with clients.

Supervisors also differ regarding the extent to which they like supervisees to prepare for supervision. Some counselling supervisors, for example, may ask their supervisees to bring tapes or transcripts of sessions with clients on a regular basis. Although this involves quite a bit of work for the supervisee, it can be immensely helpful, particularly if the supervisee is still in training.

Supervisees on their part may like to know how the supervisor goes about the supervision. You may like to know whether the supervisor uses a particular model, or whether they favour particular tools and techniques. Some supervisors are fond of using creative tools, such as art work, writing techniques or more active methods (these will be discussed in Chapter 4). However, if this is not your cup of tea, your supervisor needs to know that, so that you can agree a way of working that is comfortable for both. I like to check whether supervisees have an understanding of the supervision process and how familiar they are with concepts such as parallel process, transference or counter-transference (van Ooijen 2000:165–169). The Seven-Eyed model, for example, includes these concepts in a non-threatening way. I do not think it is essential for supervisees to have a grounding in psychodynamic theory in order to understand the significance of these phenomena in relation to supervision.

How will we ensure safety and confidentiality?

Here I would like to stress the importance of adhering to agreed boundaries. I already discussed the importance of not mixing counselling and supervision, and of keeping the managerial and the supervisory roles distinct. However, there are other boundaries that need to be attended to, such as time. Sometimes people new to supervision feel that the emphasis on time boundaries is over the top. 'What's wrong with starting 5 or 10 minutes late, going over by half an hour, or cancelling a session at short notice if you are busy?' they say. Well, I don't know about you, but I tend to plan my day in chunks of time. Therefore, if I have booked a session to last from, say, 3 until 4 o'clock in the afternoon, it is likely that my next appointment will be at 4.15 or 4.30. Going over time is therefore not an option as that would not only put out other people, but would also prevent me from writing my notes, having a break, or a cup of tea, or even making a phone call or two. So far this is just to do with good manners, I hear you say. This is undeniably true, good manners are a good idea. It is also saying in effect 'We both take the supervision seriously and we value it and each other enough to be punctual.'

Also, when we know that a session is going to last for, say, exactly 1 hour, we know what we are in for. In counselling terms it provides a container in which we can feel safe and held. Starting late is annoying if you are the one who is on time, sitting there twiddling your thumbs. Going over time when the issue being discussed is particularly interesting or difficult may seem a generous and good thing to do at the time. However, this may not at all be how the supervisee experiences it. I have been told on more than one occasion by a supervisee how angry they were with their supervisor for going over time. 'Did you not feel that they were giving you a lot of support?' I asked. No, they did not. Instead they were furious at missing their next appointment, or their bus, or they felt unsafe. 'If he keeps me for an extra half hour when we have agreed to finish at 3, I cannot help wondering what else does he not adhere to,' one person said. She felt that the supervisor's laxity with time might spill over into other areas such as confidentiality. Also, the stretching of the hour meant that she felt at sea, not knowing when they were going to finish and therefore uncertain to what extent she should engage with the process. The conclusion of all this is that maintaining appropriate boundaries needs to be taken very seriously.

How do we see accountability?

Who is accountable for what may depend on a number of factors. If the supervisee is a qualified practitioner working autonomously (such as a counsellor in private practice, for example), accountability clearly lies with the supervisee. However, if for whatever reason the supervisor becomes concerned about the practitioner's work, the supervisor is accountable for addressing it. In other words, the supervisor is accountable for the supervision. As monitoring people's work is part of the function of supervision, any concerns need to be discussed with the supervisee first. However, if, for whatever reason the supervisee refuses to acknowledge the problem, then it may be necessary for the supervisor to take action, but not without informing the supervisee first. What that action might consist of will depend on the ethical code both practitioners are working under. Having a copy of the code available is therefore a good idea.

If the supervision is part of training then the supervisor may carry more accountability for the supervisee's work, depending on the contract he or she has with the training organisation. The same goes for workplace supervision. It is important that everyone is very clear as to who is accountable for what, and it is useful for any organisation to have specific procedures in place when actions need to be taken.

How will we resolve any problems between us?

Although hopefully supervision is by and large a positive and supportive experience for most of us, we do lay our work and therefore ourselves open to scrutiny, which is not always easy. Also, by definition, those of us engaged in the helping professions work with people who are distressed in some way or another. At times this distress may affect us in ways that we are not aware of and may perhaps be unprepared for. Distress may also come into the supervision process, which, if it is spotted, can be very usefully worked with. It is useful to flag up the possibility of these kinds of problems to people new to supervision as part of the initial process of getting to know each other.

How will we know whether we are effective and working well?

It is useful to check this out at the end of every session and to give each other feedback on how the session was experienced. This will be discussed further in Chapter 6, but for now I should like to say that the clue lies in how we feel during and after a supervision session.

If, in whatever way, we feel that something is not quite right (as I did in the above example when I mixed supervision and counselling), it is important to pay attention to that feeling. All may not be well if, as a supervisor, I feel frustrated, because I think the supervisee is not listening, is defensive, or already seems to know all the answers, making me feel redundant. Alternatively, I may find myself being far too active, and stray into giving premature advice or telling the supervisee exactly what to do.

As a supervisee all may not be well if I do not feel that I am being listened to. I may feel that the supervisor does not really see me, and feel unfairly judged. Things are not going well either if I feel that the supervisor does not give me a chance to say what I am thinking or feeling before he starts giving me all kinds of advice.

When we are working well I feel clearer after a session and tend to find that the supervision is influencing how I work. My confidence will be growing and I feel that I am learning a great deal.

How long do we want to agree to work together?

Relationships are not created instantaneously but are developed over time. The people concerned have to learn to trust and respect each other and demonstrate that they are worthy of such trust and respect. Depending on how often you meet it can therefore take up to a year before both parties feel comfortable enough to be so open and trusting that challenge and probing are part of the normal way of working (Page & Wosket 2001:48). This is not to say that challenge and probing do not occur much earlier – of course they do – but there are levels to this. I think it is therefore good to potentially agree to work together for a number of years, but to review the arrangement on an annual basis. Some people like to work with the same supervisor for years on end. If the relationship is a good one and remains challenging and effective, this is fine. However, the longer people work together the more likely it becomes that things get too comfortable. Also, there may come a time when the supervisee has learnt all she has to learn from that particular supervisor. In that case, it becomes time to move on. I personally like to change my supervision arrangements every 3 to 4 years, as, no matter how good my supervisor is, I enjoy the challenge of looking for and meeting a new person with their own unique brand of knowledge and skills.

STEP 3: THE 'WHAT NOW' OF A WORKING AGREEMENT

Questions to address

- What do I think and feel Now about this person: personally? professionally?
- What else do I need to ask Now?
- What might I need to think about Now?
- What steps do we want and need to take Now?
- What goals (short- and long-term) can we Now agree?
- What can we agree on Now regarding the goals and the process of supervision?
- What are we going to commit ourselves to Now?

A written agreement is invaluable as a guide in case of problems and uncertainties. Once you both know what you have agreed, you know where you are and you can get on with the supervision. As a working agreement is the product of the negotiation between supervisor and supervisee, I find it helpful for both of us to have a signed copy of it. This is because each agreement is likely to be subtly different. Having an actual copy also means that we do not have to rely on our memory and it helps to prevent misunderstandings when we are not sure what to do or things get sticky. If the negotiation has been verbal only, there is the possibility that both parties have a slightly different interpretation of what was agreed. This can happen particularly when people are stressed or anxious, either about the supervision itself or about their work in general. A written agreement also makes it easier to review it regularly.

I believe that it is useful if both parties keep notes, perhaps in the form of a journal, not only of the process of the sessions, but also of any decisions that have been taken. The outcome of any decisions can also be jotted down in this journal, which, over time will provide a file of evidence for the effectiveness of the supervision. Note-taking is discussed in more detail in Chapter 8.

The 3-Step format can be used in the writing of the working agreement as follows:

- Step 1: What do we want to include?
- Step 2: How do we want to address these issues?
- Step 3: What do we feel Now about what we have written? Do we need to change anything?

I believe that the shorter and simpler a working agreement is, the more likely it is that it will be adhered to. Some people spend a long time on writing a really intricate and complicated document. However, when it comes to it such a document is either forgotten or does not quite address the particular issue. It is therefore easier to agree the broad principles, but leave the particulars to the practice of supervision. If problems occur both parties can refer back to the principles they have both agreed and work out how they can alter their practice to be in line.

TWO EXAMPLES OF A WORKING AGREEMENT

Example 1

The first example is brief but effective and written according to the 3-Step format (Fig. 2.1).

Working Agreement for Clinical Supervision

Between..........................the supervisee and.................................the supervisor

WHAT	HOW	WHAT NOW
Ground rules		
Place	The Pink Room 12 Pink Grove Pinktown	We agree to work together for 6 months, then evaluate using the agreed format
Dates	Alternate Tuesdays, starting.......................	
Length	11–12.30	
Cancellations	Minimum of 48 hours notice, or full fee is payable	
Holidays	We will give each other as much notice as possible	
Purpose	Honest reflection on practice to maintain and improve standard of work, helped by support and challenge	
Accountability	The supervisee is accountable for her own practice and decides what to bring to supervision	
Confidentiality	The supervisor will not take what is discussed outside the sessions, other than (occasionally) for her own supervision. In that case the supervisee will remain anonymous	

Signed..   ....
                    Supervisee   Supervisor

Date..........................2003

Figure 2.1   A brief working agreement for clinical supervision, written according to the 3-Step format.

Working Agreement for Clinical Supervision

Between.............................the supervisee and...................................the supervisor

Ground rules
  Frequency: weekly
  Length of sessions: 60 minutes
  Cancellation of sessions: minimum of 48 hours notice
  Punctuality: we agree to be punctual

Limits and boundaries
  We agree to abide by the (insert relevant Ethical Code)
  In case of a possible breach of the code we agree to discuss how to proceed
  Discussions are in confidence, other than the supervisor's own supervision
  Note-taking:
    the supervisee keeps own notes
    the supervisor keeps brief notes that are agreed with supervisee
  Boundaries of supervision:
    whereas supervision involves an exploration of the supervisee's work and her
    thoughts and feelings about the work, we understand that personal counselling
    is not part of the supervision process

Accountability
  The supervisee is accountable for her own practice
  Relationship between supervisee, supervisor and manager
  ....(insert what is appropriate)

Aims and goals
  The purpose of supervision is...
  The required balance between supportive, educational and normative function is
  ....

Responsibilities
  Agenda setting (decide whether this is determined prior to the session or
  left open)

Preferred process
  Balance between support and process is..
  Model or structure to be used is..
  Techniques that may be used include...
  Evaluation: Method to be used...............................Frequency...............................

Signed.......................................   ....
                     Supervisee   Supervisor

Date.........................2003

Figure 2.2 Working agreement of clinical supervision that would be useful for
supervision within an organisation.

Example 2

This second example (Fig. 2.2) is based on the discussion in my previous book and is useful for supervision within an organisation (van Ooijen 2000). It is more formal and includes a number of extra categories. However, I would like to encourage you to develop the agreement that feels appropriate to your situation and that you are happy with. No matter how brilliant and comprehensive an off-the-shelf document may be, it is useless if it does not fit your particular situation.

CONCLUSION

In this chapter I have discussed the skills, qualities and attitudes that are helpful for supervision. The 3-Step method was suggested as a useful framework for the initial 'getting to know each other' phase of supervision and the development of a constructive working agreement. In the next chapter I will focus on how the 3-Step method may be used to accomplish the tasks of supervision.

Questions for further reflection

- What 'groundwork' do you do before embarking on a supervisory relationship with someone?

- What advice would you give to someone who is looking for a new supervisor?

- As a result of reading this chapter, do you want to make any changes in the way you currently develop a working agreement? If so, what changes do you want to make and what are your reasons?

3

Introducing the 3-Step method of doing supervision

Supervision does not 'just happen'. (Carroll 1996:88)

 EXAMPLE

The other day I happened to be near a supermarket and thought that it would be a good idea to get the weekly shopping out of the way. I went in and bought what I thought was needed. When I came home I found to my dismay that I would have to go back as I had bought things I did not need (a third pack of oats, a second cauliflower), but still needed to restock on tea, toilet rolls and milk. As I drove back to the shop I pondered on my inefficiency and thought that if only I had applied the 3-Step supervision method to my shopping trip I would not now be going back.

In this chapter I first outline some of the tasks of supervision and explain how the 3-Step method can help to structure a clinical supervision session. The remainder of the chapter constitutes the transcript of a supervision session conducted according to the 3-Step method. I have deliberately chosen a fairly straightforward session in order to provide an overview of the method. An analysis of the session is provided in order to clarify what skills were used, what their purpose was and how they addressed the three functions of supervision.

STRUCTURING A SESSION

The 3-Step method is characterised by openness and flexibility. As it is not linked to any particular model, theoretical orientation or profession, it can be used in any helping context, irrespective of the actual profession of the worker. Together the three steps constitute a framework or structure for a session as well as a step-by-step guide on how to run it. It is therefore particularly useful for those new to supervision, although more experienced people may also find it helpful. Some authors have expressed concern at trying to define supervision, as this could lead to 'rigidity of thinking and practice' (Kelly et al in Cutcliffe et al 2001:12). The 3-Step method offers a means of counteracting such rigidity as it offers a multi-theoretical framework and a variety of methods and tools for action, for both supervisors and supervisees. So, apart from being useful in itself, the 3-Step method can incorporate more specialised models and help supervisors to tailor what they do to the needs of particular supervisees, the concerns they bring and the profession or organisation to which they belong. In short, the 3-Step method provides a structure – which includes such elements as times, place, privacy, boundaries and a thorough working agreement – within which the process of supervision can happen. Essentially, supervision is a process within a structure. The clearer and stronger the structure, the safer people will feel to engage with the process.

The idea of 'cross-over', which was first developed in relation to the Double Helix Model, is also relevant here (van Ooijen 2000:134–154). Because the 3-Step method forms a rough framework and can therefore encompass a variety of models, theories or approaches, it lends itself to be used by those who wish to 'cross-over' theoretical or professional cultures. By this I mean that supervisory couples do not necessarily have to belong to the same professional group. Such 'cross-over' will help counteract the rigidity feared by Kelly et al (in Cutcliffe et al 2001:12) and is one of the ways in which professional blind spots can be avoided.

We need structure, not just in supervision but also in life, as it gives us something to grasp hold of and so helps us to have a handle on things. People who practise yoga may find the following analogy useful. In yoga, the emphasis is on keeping the spine firm so that the internal organs can relax. If the spine is weak, the internal organs are unprotected. Similarly, in supervision the

---

Box 3.1   Properties of the 3-Step method

- Provides a framework or structure for a session
- Supervision-specific
- Simple
- Adaptable to the needs of the supervisee; such needs may involve experience, discipline, theoretical framework, context, etc.
- Can be adjusted to different professional groups
- Can incorporate any counselling approach
- Can encompass a diversity of useful methods, tools and skills
- Can be integrated with a developmental approach
- Can help make explicit the three functions of supervision (educative, supportive and monitoring)

---

structure must be firm so that the reflective process can happen. Reflection involves going back to, or deeper into, something in order to get a sense of what may be quite nebulous and difficult to get hold of. It is about creating meaning, not 'the meaning' or 'the truth', but what things mean to me, now, at this moment in time. Reflection can help me now in my imagination to go back to my work and to be in the situation with the client. A structured supervision session allows us to do that, as we know its boundaries and therefore feel safe. Without structure we would be lost, rudderless, not knowing where we are going. If the structure is weak or absent, supervisees may feel unsafe, causing part of their attention to be focused on protecting themselves.

I developed the 3-Step method as a result of realising that this is how I do in fact structure every session. Also, it is a method many of us implicitly use for everyday activities, which makes it easy to remember. Each of the three steps comprises areas that need to be addressed. However, the way in which this is done may vary, depending on the supervisee's developmental stage, experience, theoretical background, preferred way of learning and reflection and what seems appropriate at the time. Box 3.1 sets out the properties of the 3-Step method.

TASKS TO BE ADDRESSED BY THE SUPERVISOR

As far as the 3-Step method is concerned, each step comes with tasks to be attended to, as well as a range of useful skills and tools.

The tasks of supervision are what we have to do in order to fulfil its functions of support, monitoring and education. By themselves these three functions do not constitute a structure for a supervision session. It would not make sense, for example, to say, 'Right, first I will provide the supervisee with some support, then I'll monitor her work and after that I'll make sure that she goes away with something that she has leant.' They are, however, useful to bear in mind when we focus on the structure of a supervision session.

 THINKING POINT

As a supervisor, how do you see yourself fulfilling the three functions of supervision?

Table 3.1 sets out some of the tasks of supervision relative to the fulfilment of its functions. Although I have divided the tasks according to the function they address, some of tasks could be listed under more than one function. For example, I have placed

Table 3.1 Tasks of supervision in relation to their function

Support function	Monitoring function	Developmental/ educative function
Establish a good working alliance	Provide constructive criticism	Help the supervisee reflect on:
Listen	Challenge practice when necessary	• Clients – to facilitate understanding
Allow supervisee to blow-off steam	Develop clear working agreement, clear lines of accountability	• Interactions and their effectiveness
Validate good practice		• Relationship with clients
Help the supervisee to:	Monitor the supervisee's adherence to their ethical code	• Own reactions to clients
• Feel safe enough to be honest		Monitor own reactions to the material brought by supervisee
• Reflect on personal reactions and feelings	Regularly evaluate effectiveness of the supervision	
• Identify possible need for further support		Tailor supervision to the supervisee's level of experience and development
	Provide supervisee with honest feedback	

'establish a good working alliance' under the support function, as without such an alliance the supervisee is very unlikely to feel supported. However, a good working alliance is also crucial to the monitoring function, as in its absence the supervisee may well feel that she needs to hide issues of concern.

USING THE 3-STEP METHOD TO STRUCTURE A SESSION

At the beginning of this chapter I related how the 3-Step method might have helped me with my shopping trip. This is what I could have done:

- Step 1:   I want to know what I need to get from the supermarket.
- Step 2:   I check my cupboards to see what I am running low on.
            I check what I need to buy for a special dinner I am planning on Saturday evening.
- Step 3:   I write a shopping list.
            I take the list with me to the supermarket.
            I buy what I need.

As you can see it is a down-to-earth, commonsense method. Now let us apply it to a supervision session. Basically, when meeting with a supervisee I ask myself as well as the supervisee questions, which may be categorised as follows:

- Step 1:   'WHAT' – What do I need to know?
- Step 2:   'HOW' – How am I going to find out?
- Step 3:   'WHAT NOW' – What will I do Now that I have found out what I wanted to know?

Figure 3.1 shows the same process in diagrammatic form.

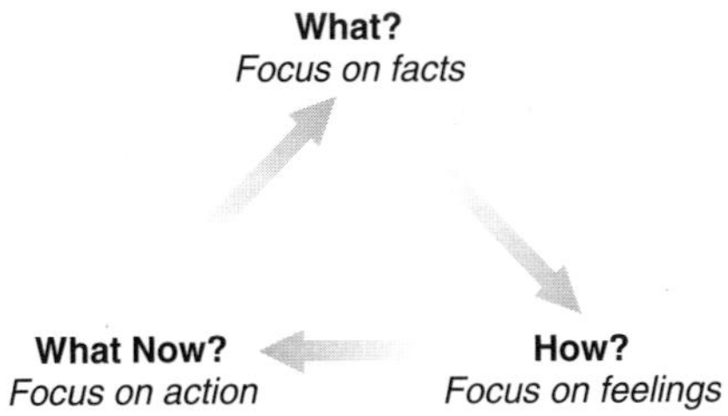

What?
Focus on facts

What Now?
Focus on action

How?
Focus on feelings

Figure 3.1   Using the 3-Step method to structure a session.

THINKING POINT

Imagine yourself in the role of supervisor. There is a supervisee sitting in front of you. He looks eager and ready to start. What kind of things will you need to know in order to help him get from the session what he needs?

STEP 1: WHAT DO I NEED TO KNOW? FOCUS ON FACTS

As a supervisor I need to know what it is that the supervisee wants to reflect on. This is not as clear-cut as it seems. As will be shown in the transcript, the supervisee may need some prompting in order to be clear on this.

The kinds of situations, relationships, events or people that supervisees want to talk about in supervision are often complicated. This makes sense as supervisees are unlikely to ask for help with something that seems straightforward, although I do believe that there is merit in examining every part of our practice, even those parts that seem unproblematic. The Greek philosopher Socrates is reported to have said, 'The unexamined life is not worth living.' Perhaps we can also add, 'The unexamined work is not worth doing', because, in the helping professions, every aspect of our work will have, either directly or indirectly, an influence on the recipients of the service that makes it worth looking at. However, complicated situations and problems tend to take precedence in supervision, which is fair enough. I have noticed that the more confusing or complicated a situation is, the less the supervisee is able to explain the situation clearly. 'I just want to talk about this,' they may say, and start talking. Ten minutes down the line, the supervisor may be equally confused and have no idea what it is that the supervisee wants from the session. This is where the supervisory skill of focusing comes in.

The 'focusing' kinds of questions I may ask are therefore along the lines of:

1. What do you want to talk about today?
2. What is your objective in doing that?
3. What do you want to achieve?
4. What is the real issue here?

Of course the situation also needs to be explained, so I may ask, 'What happened?' While listening to the answer, it is again important not to get carried away in a mass of detail, but to bear in mind the supervisee's stated objective. As supervision is a time-limited activity (an hour's session seems common), it is always a balance between allowing the supervisee to blow off steam and to get things off their chest, and helping them reflect in order to gain greater clarity. In other words, there needs to be a balance between the three functions of supervision. 'My supervisor is too supportive,' someone said to me recently. I was surprised, as to have a supportive supervisor sounds wonderful. The problem was that this was almost all that was on offer. The supervisor would listen, empathise, pat the supervisee on the back, so to speak, and say they were doing a good job. This was fine for the first few sessions. The supervisee felt respected and valued and really liked the supervisor; she felt they were building up a good relationship. After a couple of months, however, she became frustrated. 'I am not learning anything,' she said, 'and what's more I am not even sure that I believe her when she says I am doing well. How do I know that she knows what she is talking about? I feel that we never really examine anything in detail. Also, I know I am a good worker, but I am not perfect. I need help to look at the bits I am not aware of – and I know they are there.' When I asked how the sessions were structured, it appeared that this was part of the problem: there was no structure. The supervisee would talk about something, the supervisor would listen and comment on aspects that were done well, and that was it. 'Why not state what you want?' I asked. 'Your supervisor needs to know what your wants and needs are for a session; it may be worth reflecting on this before you go.'

So, the main tasks of Step 1 are first of all to help the supervisee explain the situation clearly and secondly to know what it is they want to achieve in the session. This means that we need to really listen. I would go so far as to say that the skill of active listening[1]

---

[1]Active listening involves listening and responding in such a way that the other person knows that you are listening and want to understand. Responses may be non-verbal, in the form of nodding, facial expressions and encouraging sounds like 'aha', 'hmm', 'uhm', etc. Verbal responses may involve reflection of fact or feeling, paraphrasing, summarising and questioning. (For a further discussion see van Ooijen 2000:83–87.)

is the most important one to cultivate, as without it you will not know what is going on for the supervisee.

STEP 2: HOW AM I GOING TO FIND OUT? FOCUS ON FEELINGS

Having heard the 'facts' of the situation as well as the supervisee's wants and needs, the scene is set for the main part of the supervision – the reflective space. As the supervisor I now know what the supervisee hopes to achieve in the session. Generally this involves achieving greater clarity on whatever it is they bring. So, how are we going to find this greater clarity?

 THINKING POINT

What do you feel is helpful here? How does your supervisor get you to reflect?

The kind of questions that need to be reflected on may include:

- How did you feel about what happened at the time?
- How do you feel now?
- How do you feel about your interventions and the impact on the other person or persons? How did you know?
- How would you have liked to feel?
- How would you like the other person to have felt?
- How might that have been?

I do not want to give the impression that each step is basically a set of questions; rather, the questions should be seen as a guide to what needs to be reflected on. As will be seen in the next three chapters, helping people to reflect can be done by many different methods. To some extent the flavour of Step 2 will depend on what the supervisee wants from the session. So the conduct and the focus of the 'how' depends on what is decided in Step 1. For example, a supervisee who wants to explore what may be going on under the surface of her interactions with people may benefit from a psychodynamic focus, as offered by parts of the Seven-Eyed Model (Hawkins & Shohet 2000). Supervisees with a different orientation, however, may prefer a more straightforward approach, such as the critical incident technique (see Chapter 9).

STEP 3: WHAT WILL I DO NOW THAT I HAVE FOUND OUT WHAT I WANTED TO KNOW? FOCUS ON ACTION

Steps 1 and 3 are linked. What we need to know here is whether the objectives identified in Step 1 have been achieved. If they have not, you may need to go back to Step 2. I find that people new to the role of supervisor often have a tendency to skip Step 2 and go straight to Step 3. As soon as a supervisee has outlined their problem, they may say 'Why don't you do ...', or 'Have you thought of ...', or 'What I did when I had a similar problem was ...' Often supervisees will listen politely and then answer with what I call 'Yes but'. They will say, 'Yes, but ...' and then explain why that particular solution will not work in this case. They will do that for whatever is suggested. This may seem strange, particularly when they have said that what they want is to find a solution to a problem.

 THINKING POINT

Why do you think people may engage in 'Yes but' behaviour? Have you ever done that yourself and, if so, do you know why that was?

'There should be no action without reflection.'

If you thought that "Yes but' behaviour occurs because of omitting Step 2, you are right. 'But we don't have time for that,' people often say. 'Our workload is so high, we are so pressured and supervisees come with so many problems.' Fine, I hear that. But what is the point of trying to do 'speed supervision' if it does not work? No matter how brilliant your solution, if your supervisee is not convinced, she is not going to implement it and you are in fact wasting your time. But even if she does listen, it is still not an efficient use of time.

THINKING POINT

Why not? If your supervisee is happy, does what you say, and comes back next time saying that it worked a treat, what is the problem?

The problem of overactive supervisors

There are a number of problems, but what they are depends to some extent on the individual supervisee.

Overactive supervisors create dependent supervisees

If all your supervisees have to do is to come to you with a problem, knowing that you will sort it out and tell them what to do, where is the reflection and where is the learning? You will create dependent supervisees who cannot function without you. Also, supervision will become very stressful for you as you will be carrying other people's problems as well as your own. Also, having to have all the answers all the time is stressful. Unless you are a supremely experienced and confident person, how can you be sure that you always get it right? After a while you may start having trouble sleeping at night!

It is important to remember, even in training supervision, that the trainee is the one with the client; their experience must therefore be respected. It is good for the supervisor to offer different viewpoints, but they must be linked to what the supervisee is experiencing. It is an educational principle that people learn best when new material can be integrated into their existing framework of knowledge and experience. In other words, we always need to start from where the other person is. Sometimes, in their enthusiasm and perhaps burdened by their sense of responsibility, training supervisors may forget this, and basically 'tell' the supervisee what they think is going on with the client and what should be done about it. Such supervisors may be revered as wise and charismatic, or disliked as arrogant and insensitive; the fact is that neither is helpful. It can be very scary for the supervisee to make clear to this brilliant and charismatic person just how much they are struggling. Also, by the supervisor taking such an 'autocratic' role, supervisees may not really learn as much as they could, as they feel that the supervisor has all the answers and will give them to them. I am not saying that supervisors should never impart knowledge or examples from their own experience, but that this should be done sensitively and appropriately.

Overactive supervisors create frustrated supervisees

Not everybody will become dependent. Some people, particularly the more independent, free-spirited ones, will get frustrated and angry. They will feel that you are not really doing your job. They want you to listen to them, help them reflect and become aware of what they were not seeing before, so that they can then get a sense of what they might want to do differently. They want to learn, grow and develop, and, above all, they probably want to have the freedom to make their own mistakes. If there is no space for any of this, they are likely to disregard you, go through the motions of supervision and pretend to go along with it, but in reality not take any notice. In a bid to assert their independence they may not take anything too complicated to supervision, create their own meaning out of what they experience, and only bring to supervision that which seems safe enough. Thus it is perfectly possible for a trainee (a counsellor, for example) who is in regular supervision to work in a way that the supervisor is not really aware of. If that is the case the time and money spent on supervision is wasted. You are wasting your time and they are wasting their time, but, above all, they are not having the supervision they need, which, ultimately, is to the detriment of their work. This is clearly an undesirable state of affairs, which can be avoided by the supervisor taking a step back, respecting the experience of the supervisee and their role in the co-creation of meaning.

A 'hands-off' style tends to work best with experienced people. However, as discussed in Chapter 1, the developmental stage of the supervisee should also be taken into account. Although inexperienced people need more input from the supervisor, here too it is important to help them develop insight and ideas, rather than just giving them the answers. So the rule is: facilitate reflection and only provide help, suggestions or information if the supervisee does not have enough experience to get there herself.

Moving on

If, after having spent time on Step 2, it is likely that the objectives identified in Step 1 have been achieved and the supervisee feels clearer, it is time to move on. The supervisee can be helped to identify what she has learnt, what she now sees differently and what, if anything, she may wish to do as a result. It is also good practice to give each other feedback on the session, what worked well, what did not work well and what, if anything, you might like to do differently next time. So the kind of questions that need to be addressed include:

- What Now do you think and feel about it?
- What Now have you learnt?
- What Now do you plan to do?

So Step 3 is about consolidation of the supervision and helping the supervisee to take this 'vision' forwards.

TRANSCRIPT OF A SUPERVISION SESSION

CONTEXT

Sonia is a social worker who has contracted to see me privately once a month. Like most social workers, she also receives supervision from her manager. However, because of workload and time constraints this is not as regular as she would like. Also, because the supervision is managerial, organisational constraints mean that the focus is on the clients rather than on Sonia. What Sonia wants from me is a place where she can use the supervision for her supportive and developmental needs, as the monitoring function of supervision is already taken care of by her manager. We have not worked together for very long, so I am not yet familiar with how she works.

During this session the interaction was sometimes punctuated with non-verbal encouragers from the supervisor such as 'umm'. For the sake of readability, most of those utterances have been eliminated from this text.

THE SESSION
Step 1: the 'what' section

Els: Hi Sonia, how would you like to use this session?
         Commentary: greeting, open question. Purpose: build
         relationship; encourage Sonia to state her aim.

Sonia: Well, there are two of my cases that I would like to talk
         about.

Els: And, how much time do you think you need for each?
         Commentary: open question. Purpose: to agree a 'mini'
         contract for the session.

Sonia: Uhm, I think about 25 minutes each. Yes, let's say
         25 minutes each, so that will leave a bit of leeway at the end.

Els: That sounds good. Leaving a bit of space at the end will give
         us a chance to reflect on how the supervision itself went.
         Commentary: supportive statement. Purpose: agreeing and
         further clarifying 'mini' contract.

Sonia: Yes, that's right. I do find that helpful. So if I can start with the
         first case. It is about an older man, I saw the other day, who
         has suddenly started to beat up his wife; he had never done
         that before. I am feeling a bit uncomfortable so I'd like to talk
         about it a bit.

Els: I am wondering what it is that concerns you?
         Commentary: open question. Purpose: focusing in on
         Sonia's aims and goals.

Sonia: I think it is about ... it is something about imposing values of
         society on people that I am concerned about. The couple
         here have lived together for over 50 years. They've had
         an absolutely fine marriage, there has been no input from
         any department or anywhere else, they have two children,
         a nice house, nicely furnished, and warmly clothed and well,
         and up to now they have not had any difficulty at all.

Els: So they are quite well physically?
         Commentary: clarifying question.

Sonia: Yes, they are both healthy, both well, mobile, they go to the
         shops, using the buses ... uhm ... She has quite a wide social

network, he has no network. He enjoys the garden, he does that. Then all of a sudden, in comes the Social Services department.

Els: So suddenly you became involved? Tell me a bit about that.
Commentary: clarifying question, verbal encourager.

Sonia: What happened was that he suddenly started to beat up his wife. The person who asked us to become involved was actually his daughter. He was hitting at his wife. The husband was distraught.

Els: He was distraught?
Commentary: reflection, encouraging comment.

Sonia: He was distraught, more distraught than she was actually ... he seemed to be unable to stop it ...

Els: So something appears to be quite out of control and at the daughter's request you went to see him ... Was this at the request of her father?
Commentary: reflection, closed, clarifying question.

Sonia: Uhm, I don't think she had much of a relationship with her father that they can talk about things ... she had a close relationship with her mother, they go out shopping and so on, but not with her father. I think she saw them quite regularly, but he tended to be a bit in the background, pottering in his garden, or tinkering with some DIY.

Els: Tell me a bit about what happened when you first went to see them. So the Social Services were contacted, you were asked to see them. So tell me a bit about that, how that went, that first contact.
Commentary: open question. Reflection. Open question.
Purpose: to encourage Sonia to explain what happened – the facts.

Sonia: When I went in, he was on his own.

Els: I see.
Commentary: encouraging comment.

Sonia: The crisis at this point had passed; it had already been sorted out by the housing department ... they had declared that she was homeless and put her into a hostel, so they had found somewhere for his wife to stay temporarily. So th. crisis, the place of safety, had already been established. . was on the Friday night; she had been there all weekend anu I went in to see him on the following Monday. I went in to see this older man, who was just completely emotionally wrung out ... he moved around very slowly, sat down in the corner ... he was almost fetal like, huddled in a corner, and all I could describe it as is as a mass of shame.

Els: Could you show me how he sat? When you said fetal like, and a mass of shame ... could you show me physically how he sat? How that was?
Commentary: closed question. Purpose: at this stage things feel rather abstract for me. Although the story is distressing I am not getting a sense of it. By asking Sonia to take up his position I am hoping that she will get more engaged with the feelings, and that I will therefore be able to picture the situation.

Sonia: He was very hunched up ... (bending her head forward and clasping her knees with her hands).

Els: All hunched up ...
Commentary: reflection. Purpose: to encourage, in effect saying 'I am listening, go on.'

Sonia: Very hunched up, head right down, not holding his head up at all, very much in posture of shame (bends her head down low over her knees).

Els: Uhm, literally hanging his head.
Commentary: reflection.

Sonia: Yes, literally hanging his head in shame; it was as if his world had come to an end.

Els: Uhm.
Commentary: non-verbal encourager.

Sonia: Which it had done ... because this was behaviour that he just never, he had never done anything like this ... he got to nearly 80 ... he had never been violent to his wife ... treating her respectfully.

Els: Can you say a bit more?
Commentary: encouraging question.

Sonia: Giving her a good family home, they are respected in the local community; they were very involved with the local church. He used to be a senior accountant, or something, for a large manufacturing firm, quite a well paid job I believe, very well respected generally, you know, respect and status … But actually, it was more about what was going on inside … about what was going on inside him.

Els: So if I can just check this out … so what you are saying is that here is a respectable couple, they appear to have had a good marriage, he is from a good background, good job and then this appears to have happened suddenly, out of the blue and out of character.
Commentary: reflection. Purpose: to check and clarify understanding.

Sonia: Yes, that is right.

Els: So the crisis was over the weekend, and his wife was taken to a place of safety and you went in on the Monday
Commentary: mini summary. Purpose: to check, first, that I have understood and, second, to help Sonia to be clearer.

Sonia: Right, yeah. My role, I would say, was in finding out what had happened and why.

Els: Right.
Commentary: verbal encourager.

Sonia: There was no suggestion that he … he did not talk about it easily … he was not answering any questions easily, he was very monosyllabic in his replies … he did not really want to talk … but there was no question of him denying what had happened. It was clear from his behaviour, you know, and the fact that he had opened the door to me, and that he had let me in.

Els: I see.
Commentary: encouraging comment.

Sonia: And we established that his wife was not there, that she was in a hostel … so the first task was to try and get him to talk about what had actually happened … and to see how it compared to what we had heard from her … obviously, because the effect it had had on her.

Els: Right ... and regarding today's session, what is it you would like to achieve as a result of talking about it?
Commentary: open, 'focusing' question. Purpose: to help Sonia become clear on what she wants from the session, as this is not yet clear.

Sonia: Well, one of the things that came across was his shame ... about Social Services ... To unravel that a bit really ... How we get involved, how the Department gets involved, and things go awry. Uhm. Almost as if we are coming along with a heavy stick, although there was no legislation that would allow us to do anything really, except to make sure that she was in a place of safety. The Housing Department had actually already taken care of that, of that initial task so it was about helping people but also establishing that this was not appropriate behaviour.

Els: So are you saying that you are feeling somewhat uncomfortable with the position that you are in ... although it was necessary and nothing else could have been done, at the same time it feels a bit heavy-handed. I don't know, is that what you are saying? Is that what you want to look at today?
Commentary: mini summary, followed by a 'focusing' question, so that we can move on to Step 2.

Sonia: Uhm, yeah ... I mean, I know that by my being there ... it has the potential of helping him ... it has the potential of helping him to unravel, however, within care management my role is to go in, to make an assessment and to go back out again. And I would assess that this couple needs some counselling-type mediation. The Department now is very much about providing and commissioning care instead of the intensive work that I think he needs in order to find out what happened.
Commentary: agrees with the aim and focus and beginning to reflect.

Els: When you say commissioning care, what do you mean?
Commentary: clarifying question.

Sonia: Arranging care providers, rather than providing care.

Els: Buying in counsellors?
Commentary: clarifying question.

Sonia: Buying in counsellors, to get counsellors.

Step 2: the 'how' section

Els: You feel, it feels like you are saying ... because ... I sense a
        lot of empathy regarding this man that this happened, and of
        course it is not a good thing, he is hanging his head in
        shame, and you feel that potentially you would like to work
        with him and provide a counselling role, either yourself or a
        colleague to find out what has happened, to sort things out
        between them – and that appears not possible with how the
        Department functions?
        *Commentary: mini summary. Clarifying question. Purpose: to
        encourage Sonia to begin to reflect on the situation.*

Sonia: It would be very difficult for me to get the time to do that. My
        feeling is that relationship building takes time, and this ... we
        have made a start and ... we could get to the bottom of
        what ... but because the Department now works in a very
        different way my role is as an assessor. And my assessment
        would be that this couple would need ... I know it would be
        strange, a stranger coming into his house, his life, and it
        would be forced. I don't think that he would initially agree to
        that, he certainly has not agreed to it at the moment. At the
        moment he has agreed to the help with the crisis, we are
        using a crisis intervention model, which means that I could
        actually work with him.
        *Commentary: beginning to reflect on the situation, imagining
        what the situation might feel like for the clients.*

Els: I suppose what I am trying to understand is how are you left
        feeling in all this because you have gone in, you will make an
        assessment – or you know what your assessment will be, that
        they need counselling. And you also know that you are not in a
        position to provide it yourself because of the way in which the
        Department is now structured. And is that really the right thing
        to do – yet another set of people to go and see them.
        *Commentary: self-disclosure – reflection. Purpose: to check
        that I understand correctly and to encourage further reflection.*

Sonia: Uhm.

Els: So how are you left feeling in all this?
        *Commentary: open question, encouraging Sonia to reflect
        on her feelings.*

Sonia: Dissatisfied. I feel that I have been called in to assist, and I have the skills and tools to do that, but because of policy and legislation now I am not being allowed to do that. Of course, I could look at it differently and in asking for specialist help I am doing something ...

Els: So what is it ... uhm ... of course you could ask for special permission, but I guess you would not do that for every person you go and see? So there is something different here, and the fact that you have brought him today suggests that there is something that needs exploring. What do you think? *Commentary: clarifying question; confrontation; closed question. Purpose: focusing on what the issue really is, deeper reflection.*

Sonia: The difference is that this man has gone through his life without any help, he has managed very well to run a house and family, he has managed to have a good relationship with his family, and that to reach an age when he would be ... My personal belief is ... he should be having respect ... I feel that if one small piece of work that could be a quality piece of work with him and his wife ... would mean that he may not need our help again, enabling him to carry on. The alternative would be that he is then in the hands of the authorities, mental health departments, social services, continuing ad infinitum.

Els: What strikes me, we are talking about him and the kind of things that might happen and how uncomfortable the situation is. And I suppose in a way both you and your client also are stuck within the situation as it is and the way things are organised.
Commentary: self-disclosure; clarifying; empathic statement.

But what I am not getting much of a sense of is how it was to be in the room with him. You say he was in a fetal position, he answered very monosyllabically, but I am getting not much of a sense of what it was like when you were with him. *Commentary: confrontation. Purpose: to help Sonia reflect more deeply.*

Sonia: I think he had become childlike and I had become mothering. I felt his shame, I felt empathy for him and wanted to protect him. Interesting that I had not actually been involved with his wife up to this point. She was in a place of safety, but at that particular point I felt that he needed protecting, from himself almost. Have someone care for him.

Els: Uhm, uhm ... so you felt quite protective.
        Commentary: reflection. Purpose: encouraging, empathy.

Sonia: Yeah, I did, yes.

Els: Hmmm, I get the feeling, uhm ...you appear to feel very strongly for this man and I find myself wondering whether it is pushing any buttons for you personally...you don't have to say if you don't want to.
        Commentary: probing. To separate out anything personal from the professional.

Sonia: Uhm, that is interesting ... yes ... yes there is something ... I had not made that connection before. It's not so much about me as about something it reminds me of. There was a situation a long time ago, when I had only just qualified ... I was very unhappy with how things were handled, but it wasn't my decision to be made. And to be honest, what I wanted to do at the time would probably not have been appropriate ... I thought I knew it all, but actually I was only just beginning.

Els: I see, so there is something in what we are talking about today that is similar?
        Commentary: probing question. Encouraging Sonia to reflect further.

Sonia: Yes, I suppose, hmm, I need to think about this a bit.

Els: I find myself wondering whether to look at this other situation for a bit, or whether that would take us away from things.
        Commentary: self-disclosure, thinking aloud. Reminder that supervision is a mutual endeavour, also giving the supervisee the option to decide what would be helpful.

Sonia: Uhm, actually, I think I'm all right. Luckily I did have good supervision at the time. What I learnt, actually, was that sometimes I get a bit overinvolved and I forget that there is usually more than one way of looking at the same situation.

Els: Yes, that is right, that sounds like an important realisation. What about this situation? What about the man? How do you think he felt about you being there?
Commentary: reflection, validation of supervisee's learning; supportive. Open question, getting Sonia to reflect on client's perspective.

Sonia: I think he responded to me, uhm, I think he also felt that he needed some help but he did not know how to get it or what it would be, or how to ask for it. If he had asked for it, it could have been weeks before, when whatever prompted this was happening.

Els: So when you say that you feel that he felt that he needed help, can you tell me what led you to that conclusion? How did you know that?
Commentary: open question. Purpose: to challenge any possible assumptions.

Sonia: Well, my experience of people who do not want to work with you, they will get up and walk if they are able to.

Els: Literally walk out of the door?
Commentary: reflection. Purpose: to encourage Sonia to say more.

Sonia: Yes, they will walk out of the door, or not answer…The fact that he was answering at all, even though it was only monosyllabically, uhm, means that he was actually engaging in something … uhm … His body language did actually relax slightly towards the end of the session that I had with him and he was OK about me coming back again.

Els: You asked him?
Commentary: clarifying question. Purpose: to make sure that this was not an assumption on Sonia's part.

Sonia: Yes, I asked him if he would like me to come back to see him again and he was OK with that. That meant to me – he could have said no thank you, or nothing at all. If he had said nothing at all I would have taken that as a no thank you too. But I got the impression that he was accepting of what I might be able to help him with.

Els: So your experience is that if people really do not want to see you again they let you know … and I guess in your experience you are able to pick up those signs of people, from what they are saying or from what they are not saying. So…you have made an assessment, you may … and you have not done that yet.

Sonia: No.

Els: So how has this left you feeling now?
Commentary: open question. Focusing in on Sonia's feelings, consolidation – relating it back to her aims as stated in Step 1 – beginning to move towards Step 3.

Sonia: It has left me feeling that I would like to do some work with him and possibly with his wife. I have not met her, I am going to see her tomorrow. Possibly at the weekend, she may be going home. She has not got any physical needs, she is well, she has seen her GP, she has no physical needs apart from the change in her husband, which is an emotional need.

Els: But you have not seen her yet … so it is very hard to know what the situation is I guess.
Commentary: confrontation. Reminding Sonia of the reality of the situation – that she only knows half the story. Any planned action needs to take this into account.

Step 3: the 'now what' section

Sonia: That is right, it is the feedback I have had from other professionals, from the duty social worker … so I have taken their assessment about her circumstances … I am more concerned about him at the moment. I would like to do a piece of work with him and how am I going to get that agreed within this system that we have?

Els: So now you need to spend a chunk of time working through the emotional situation? And you feel that is something you would really like to do?
Commentary: reflective question. Checking out Sonia's wishes for action.

Sonia: Yes.

Els: And the alternative is?

Commentary: open question. To look the planned action from all angles.

Sonia: The alternative is … eh, complete the assessment with the wife obviously. But at the end of the day – if there are no other needs, withdraw. There are no physical needs, and if there is no need for a place of safety, ehm … the potential may be that we do not get involved again and that everything is sorted.

Els: Right, so literally it is crisis intervention. Something happened, he became violent towards his wife and the daughter asked for help, so that was the immediate problem, his wife had to be in safety, what you say could happen is that if things appear to have calmed down, his wife will come home again and that is what will happen.
Commentary: mini summary. To check out that it has all been understood correctly – then to consolidate, to help Sonia to move on.

Sonia: It may be that everything is nicely capped. And it may be that it will not happen again. But also there is a possibility that he may do this again or he actually becomes very insular. His confidence has gone completely, because of his loss of self-esteem, his loss of control, he may even potentially be a mental health services user in the future.

Els: So what you seem to be saying is, if I do some work with him now then it might prevent it happening again or it might prevent it having an adverse effect on his mental health. I see, I understand it better now. But on the other hand, if the assessment is that they both appear all right now and there is no immediate need then that kind of help may not be available.
Commentary: summary. To check understanding and to help Sonia to move on.

Sonia: Yes, that is right.

Els: And that is your responsibility? To make that kind of assessment? Is that right?
Commentary: closed question. To check both my understanding and that Sonia is doing the right thing.

Sonia: That is right make that assessment and make the argument with my manager as to the way forward.

Els: And at the moment you have a lot of empathy with him, but of course we only have half the story so far. We don't know yet what his wife will say. Do you have any fantasies about that?
Commentary: reflection. Confrontation. Support plus focusing on the 'unknown' part of the scenario.

Sonia: I think she will say that everything is fine. That it was a one-off, and I will go home and everything will be fine. I do not anticipate her saying I feel threatened and unsafe and I want to move out permanently.

Els: Uhm, uhm. And how would that be, if that is what she said?
Commentary: open question. To help Sonia be clear and to plan her actions.

Sonia: Without working it through it is going to make a change to their relationship. Their relationship is such that he has at least an equal part to play in their relationship. I figure that one possibility may be that she may be more wary in that relationship or she smothers him with love and does not allow him to do anything. Both of which will be detrimental to the future.

Els: So what you appear to be saying is … you would like it to be looked into.
Commentary: reflection. To help Sonia be clear.

Sonia: I would like to be given the time to do that piece of work with him and possibly her too.

Els: And do you think that is likely?
Commentary: closed question. To focus Sonia on the reality and help plan action.

Sonia: Not unless I put a very good argument over …

Els: And what would be your fall-back position? If your manager says, well Sonia you have a heavy workload already and …this is going to be to the detriment of all this other work that you need to be doing, what would your answer to that be?
Commentary: open question. Supportive challenge. Help Sonia plan her action in more detail.

Sonia: As I said, there is the potential for using the … services, the potential of a long-term cost of care is greater than the short-term cost.

Els: So that would be quite a good argument. But what you were saying earlier was that they need counselling, but that that kind of work needs to be contracted out, so I am just wondering about that.
        Commentary: reflection. Confrontation and clarification.

Sonia: The other aspect is the time of when it is needed. It is not needed in 6 months, or 3 years, it is needed now.

Els: And if it was contracted out?

Sonia: Yes, if it was successfully contracted out … and it is not a priority need … it could take up to 6 months before they were seen by anyone.

Els: So you seem to be clear on what you would like to happen.
        Commentary: reflection. Supportive.

Sonia: I suppose I am, now. (Laughs) I am now much clearer regarding how I feel and what I want to do. As you say, I'll see his wife and then I decide what to do. If it does seem that they would benefit from help now I will make a good case to my manager. Particularly the cost element might be quite persuasive.

Els: That sounds good. We have almost come to the end of the 25 minutes. Is there anything else on this?
        Commentary: reminder of the working agreement.

Sonia: No, that feels good. Yes, right, let me just think of my next case …

And so on.

The above transcript represents part of a fairly straightforward supervision session. The supervisee had prepared in that she knew what she wanted to bring. However, she was unclear as to exactly what she wanted. It seemed that her feelings of discomfort got in the way of clarity and I had to keep going back to the question 'What is it you need from this session?' This often happens.

All the supervisee may know is that they feel stuck, or confused or uncomfortable. It is the job of the supervisor to help the supervisee to focus in on what she wants and needs, so that there will be a specific outcome to the session. As will be discussed in Chapter 7, it is a good idea to make a note of the agreed outcomes, as it is one of the ways in which the effectiveness of the supervision can be evaluated.

CONCLUSION

In this chapter I introduced the 3-Step method to structuring a supervision session. In the following four chapters I will examine each step in greater detail and offer a range of helpful tools and techniques.

Questions for further reflection

- Do you want to make any changes in the way you currently structure your supervision sessions?

- What changes do you want to make?

- What are your reasons for wanting to do so?

- What do you think of 'overactive' supervisors?

4

Beginning supervision: working with the 'what' section

Begin with the end in mind. (Covey 1992:145)

In this chapter, I first focus on the importance of further developing the working alliance, which includes paying attention to people's previous experiences of supervision and what they have learnt from it. Next, the skills, qualities and tasks associated with Step 1 are further elaborated and discussed with relevance to the supervisor as well as the supervisee.

DEVELOPING THE WORKING ALLIANCE

For the supervisor, the overarching question here is: 'What do I want to know?'

 THINKING POINT

Just imagine you have had your initial meeting or meetings with each other and have developed a working agreement. Now it is your first real supervision session. First, as a supervisor, what is it you want to know about the supervisee? Then, as a supervisee, what would you like the other person to know?

As a supervisor, once I start working with someone I like to find out more about the person as well as her work. In the first few sessions I find it helpful to build further on the 'getting to know each other' conversation we began at our initial meeting, as we need to get used to each other and our ways of working.

THE IMPORTANCE OF PAYING ATTENTION TO THE WORKING ALLIANCE

Although in the first session we have spent time getting to know each other and have drawn up a working agreement, we do not as yet have a solid working alliance. That takes time and has to be earned, from both sides. A number of studies have shown that counsellors preferred supervisors' primary focus to be the relationship rather than the task (Usher & Borders 1993, Webb & Wheeler 1998). Unless the supervisee brings a particular issue that she really wants to work on, I may therefore encourage her to talk about herself in relation to her work in more general terms. For example, I may say:

• Tell me about your work.
• What do you feel you are doing well?
• What are your areas of difficulties?
• Where do you see yourself in your development as a practitioner?
• How would you describe yourself as a practitioner?
• How do you think others might describe you?
• How would you like to be talked about?

Supervisees often find these questions very interesting as it helps them to look at their work afresh and to highlight some areas that need further consideration. When I am in the role of supervisee I really want my supervisor to ask these questions as I feel that they need to know me as a person as well as a professional. Being facilitated to reflect in this way makes me feel that here is a person who is really interested in me as well as in what I do.

The supervisee's previous experience of supervision can also be further elaborated. I find it helpful to know what worked for them and what did not, as it may indicate areas of possible future difficulties. To be forewarned is to be forearmed, and that goes for both of us. If a particular previous experience was difficult it may be useful to explore this a bit. I like to know what it was that was difficult and what prevented it from being a positive learning experience. Sometimes processes and situations need to be repeated several times before we are able to learn what there is to learn. So it may well be that a similar difficult situation will occur again. Only this time we can both be on the lookout for it so we can then name what is going on. In other words, rather than getting stuck in the difficulty, we can both own our part in it and find a way through it together. But even if previous experiences of supervision have been nothing but positive, supervisees are always likely to be somewhat wary when coming to a new one (Bramley 1996:37).

So, at the beginning of the supervision relationship there is a need to get used to each other. It would be unreasonable for me to expect a supervisee to be as open and honest in the first or second session as when we have been working together for a year. Particularly in the health professions, where people may not have been used to reflecting on their own feelings, a question such as 'What are you feeling about that?' may well get answered by what they are thinking. Sometimes there is blank incomprehension: 'What do you mean what I am feeling? I have already said that I think that it was … etc.' Now, what I want to say about such defensiveness is that first of all the supervisee may not be conscious of it and secondly that it does have a value as we defend ourselves for a reason. We defend ourselves when we feel under threat of attack or annihilation (as in war, for example). Something similar is at work in the helping professions as at an unconscious level we may feel under assault from some kind of distress, the cause of which may be physical illness or mental, emotional or social distress or a combination of any or all of these. Working with the distressed is not easy and to some extent we may therefore feel that we need to protect ourselves. Such protection is expressed by, for example, a rigid emphasis on rules and procedures, on maintaining a strict professional distance, or on simply not really engaging with any of it at a real level. The trouble with these defensive strategies is that they are only successful up to a point. Even if we are not aware of it consciously, we are affected by the distress – it does go in somewhere.

Rather than regarding this as something bad or unprofessional, it is good to recognise it. After all, it is happening, so it is not useful to stick our heads in the sand. But this then begs the question of how can we help ourselves to cope with it. And, perhaps more radically, we might even begin to wonder whether being affected by our clients might actually be helpful and assist us in becoming even better practitioners. I believe that the answer is yes, but only with help, or eventually we will get burnt out. Clinical supervision is an ideal vehicle for looking at how our clients affect us, either consciously or unconsciously. Good supervision can be very supportive in discharging some of the unavoidable distress. It can help us unravel our feelings about our clients and develop ways in which we can usefully work with them. (How this can be done will be discussed further in the next chapter.) However, this means that not only do supervisors need to be trained, they also need to know what it is like to have this kind of supervision for themselves. In an ideal world, we would all have supervision from the moment we start working in our chosen profession. In addition, experienced people should be encouraged to undergo supervision training so that there need never be a shortage of supervisors. If this becomes the status quo – a way in which we in the helping professions help ourselves to help our clients – I believe that there will be far less turnover and burnout and that as a result we will be much more effective in helping our clients.

THE STAGES OF LEARNING

I also like to know what worked particularly well and how aware supervisees are about how they learn best. You may be aware of the stages we go through in becoming competent at something. First we are unconsciously incompetent, then we become consciously incompetent, followed by conscious competence and finally unconscious competence. What can often happen in supervision is that people's unconscious incompetence gets illuminated, thus making it conscious. This is very uncomfortable and many people want to rush past this stage. By the way, this goes for the supervisor as well as the supervisee. If you are a new supervisor, you are likely to be at the stage of conscious incompetence. If that is the case, brilliant. You and your supervisees can have a working agreement that recognises that conscious incompetence is a good experience to have. In fact, it is a necessary experience! Realising that this stage is essential and cannot be jumped can help make this stage less frustrating. You and your supervisees can learn together; in fact, it is often a very good learning experience for supervisees too. Also consciously engaging with the stage provides excellent role modelling! If we do try and jump straight from unconscious incompetence to conscious competence, guess what will happen? Sooner or later, we will fall and hurt ourselves. And the higher we have jumped, the harder we will fall.

ROLE-MODELLING

In fact, the role model aspect of supervision should not be over-looked. By virtue of the fact that we have agreed to function as a supervisor, we implicitly take on some authority. I think this is always the case, even with peers. This does not mean that super-visors need to tell supervisees what to do. Rather it means that they own their knowledge and experience, and speak and act from that. So if, for example, something in the supervision rela-tionship is not working, or feels uncomfortable, it is important that the supervisor brings it out into the open. If this is not done, it is basically saying to the supervisee 'It is OK to avoid difficult issues.' A supervisor who abdicates her authority like that is likely to engage in collusive behaviour and effectively teach the super-visee to do the same. Conversely, supervisors who are too quick to jump on any perceived shortcoming, perhaps before they have heard the whole story, will have the effect of supervisees editing what to bring. Unfortunately, it is likely that what is being edited also happens to be the very thing that needs to be looked at!

 EXAMPLE

A counsellor had a problem in sticking to time boundaries with a particular client. As soon as she mentioned that she had let a session overrun on a number of occasions, her supervisor interrupted and proceeded to give her a lecture on the importance of sticking to time boundaries and gave her some strategies for doing so. This was not what the counsellor needed, as it was exactly her awareness of the importance of sticking to time boundaries that had prompted her to bring it as a problem to supervision in the first place. What she wanted was an exploration of the dynamics between her and her client that made this so difficult. Being lectured, however, left her angry and unwilling to engage with the issue further as she feared being judged even more. 'I just did not feel safe anymore,' she told me.

This example may be described as a break in the supervisory rela-tionship and, like any break, it depends on its size and whether it was a first or subsequent break as to whether reparation is possible. The counsellor was able to address the issue in a subsequent session, which led to a frank discussion between her and her supervisor. Although clearly this was not comfortable for the supervisor, he appreciated the supervisee bringing it up and they had an honest and frank discussion as to how each of them felt they were relating to each other. This cleared the air and paved the way for the counsellor to explore how she and her client were relating in turn. In effect, the supervisor had role-modelled a willingness to engage with something uncomfortable and an openness to looking at his own way of working. The fact that they had discussed the possibility of this kind of thing happening in the working agreement and agreed ways of dealing with it was also very helpful.

THE IMPORTANCE OF STEP 1

The problem that occurred in the above example could have been avoided if the beginning of the session had been given more attention. It seemed that the supervisor did not have a structure and was not in a habit of asking supervisees for their goals of a session. If he had done so the session might have run very differently. The beginning might have been along the following lines:

Supervisee: I would like to talk about client A. There is something going on between us, and I don't know what it is.

Supervisor: Say a bit more?

Supervisee: Well, it is becoming very difficult to end the sessions on time, in fact, I have overrun by 5 minutes three times now.

Supervisor: And how are you normally regarding time boundaries?

Supervisee: I am normally fine; it is just with this particular client that my best intentions seem to go to pot.

Supervisor: I see. So what you are saying is that you feel that there is something going on here that is different?

Supervisee: Yes, that is right and I would like to explore what it is. Somehow it feels really significant.

In this alternative scenario, all that happened was that the supervisor gave the supervisee a bit of space so that she herself identified the focus as well as the goal of the session: to explore the phenomenon going on and to find out what dynamics are at play.

FOCUS ON FACTS

There are no facts without frameworks, no data without meaning. (Hobson 1985:xii)

In order to identify the supervision question it is necessary to hear some facts first. Who is the client or what is the situation, what happened, what did you do, etc. are all valid questions to ask during this process. However, without a framework within which to place the facts, they would get lost. As the above example shows, the facts told by the supervisee were the same, but the meaning to her of those facts – that they were significant and needed exploring – only came to light once there was a framework within which they could be placed.

THE VALUE OF MISTAKES

As the above example indicates, mistakes in supervision can be very valuable. The working alliance has to be strong enough though and the supervision space safe enough. If both of these are in place, supervisor and supervisee can talk about what has been going on undefensively and explore what the reasons for it might be. Supervisors will do their supervisees a great service if they can model this way of working. For example, if a supervisor has made a mistake (perhaps uncharacteristically giving premature advice, or forgetting something important), he could say, 'I have made a mistake, that is interesting. Let's look at what happened.' This kind of supervisor, who is not afraid to own mistakes but has an attitude of curiosity and interest, is likely to foster the same kind of attitude in his supervisees. Now contrast this with the supervisor who will never do so, instead pretending that it did not happen. The unspoken message here is that mistakes are shameful, that the one who made them may be judged harshly and that therefore mistakes should be hidden at all cost.

Mistakes as learning opportunities

Recently I took a course with Babette Rothschild. Before sending us off to practise something she had just taught us, she would encourage us not to be afraid, but to go away and make lots of mistakes. When we came back, she would ask, 'Who has made any mistakes?' And then, 'Oh good, that means that you are really learning.' Her point was that we learn best through making mistakes. She used to say (Rothschild 2000), 'If you already know everything, what are you doing here? You should be in my place.'

So mistakes, whether made by supervisors or supervisees, should be seen as providing us with valuable opportunities for learning. I like to think of mistakes as mis/takes. You have probably seen what happens when people make a film. The scene is set, the actors are ready, someone brings down the lever on the clapperboard and says 'take 53', or whatever. No matter how good the actors or how experienced the film-maker, it is extremely rare for the first 'take' to be the one that is kept. If talented and experienced people find it necessary and useful to do the same thing again and again, why should the rest of us worry if we may not get it right first time? Also, I do not think that getting it right first time is always a good thing. As far as supervision is concerned, you may do a really good session with someone, but when asked afterwards what it was that you did you may not necessarily know. And, if you don't know what you did or how you did it, you may not be able to repeat it. In other words, you may not have learnt from it. Now, it is a funny thing about mistakes, but somehow they stick in our minds much more than the things we get right, which is what makes them such ideal learning opportunities (Box 4.1).

Having just extolled the virtues of mistakes, I do want to point out a few common ones that it would be good to avoid:

- Not listening (the pre-occupied supervisor).
- Following own agenda (the supervisor thinks she knows best).
- Premature advice (the supervisor who leaves out Step 2).
- Being 'too' knowledgeable (the supervisor who does not facilitate the learning of her supervisee).

Box 4.1 A 'mis/take' is a learning opportunity

Getting it right first 'take' is not always ideal because:

- You may not know how you did it
- You will not know how to do it again

It is not a hanging offence if you do, occasionally, find yourself making some of the above mistakes. I know I do. But, as mentioned earlier, what would be unhelpful is to then pretend that it did not happen. Creating a learning opportunity out of the mistake involves first of all owning up to it, and secondly to look at why it happened.

THE SKILLS, QUALITIES AND TASKS OF STEP 1

Remember BABE

BABE is an acronym of four helpful qualities in the avoidance of mistakes (in memory of that little pig in the eponymous film that made its way in the world):

Be yourself
Awake, aware, alert
Be prepared
Evaluate

TASKS, SKILLS, QUALITIES AND METHODS

The start of every session is like a mini working agreement regarding its goals and tasks (Gilbert & Evans 2000:68). The main task at Step 1 therefore involves helping the supervisee to be clear on what it is she wants from the supervision session. However, supervision needs the active involvement by both supervisor and supervisee as is clear from Table 4.1.

Tasks

Starting a session

Before even asking supervisees what they want to talk about I think it is a good idea to have a 'check-in' time of, say, 5 or 10 minutes. Bramley calls it 'emergency time', which can be used to arrive in the room, as it were. People may have rushed to get there, or had a bit of a journey, or have just come out of a tricky situation. Setting some time aside at the beginning allows for any left-over feelings to be discharged and shared. This time can also be used for any general questions the supervisee may have or any discussions regarding changes in the agreed dates, perhaps because of

Table 4.1 Step 1: the 'what' section

	Supervisor	Supervisee

Tasks	Use of time
	Clarity re topic
	Identify desired outcomes
	   and learning objectives
		Select topic
		Identify needs, wants,
		   hopes and fears

Qualities	Openness Relationship building Comfortable with 'not knowing' Attitude of respectful curiosity	Openness Relationship building Honesty Ability to trust

Skills	Active listening
	(Help supervisee describe,
	   summarise and focus)
	Questioning
	Analysis
		Describe
		Able to engage with
		   questions

Methods, tools, techniques	Prepare
	Questioning
	Scene-setting
	Role-play
	Use of props
	Drawing
	Writing and other
	   creative methods
		Prepare
		Select from reflective log
		Quiet space – reflection
		   before the session

forthcoming holidays. Once all this is out of the way it leaves the rest of the session free to be used productively.

Use of time

In Step 1 the scene is set for the whole session, so it is important to get it right. The main task therefore involves an agreement on how to use the time. For example, in the example in Chapter 3 the supervisee wanted to bring two issues. If the supervisor had not asked her how much time she thought she might need for each, the first issue might have taken up a disproportionate amount of time, thus not leaving enough space for the second one. It is the task of the supervisor to monitor the use of time, as expecting the supervisee to do so may get in the way of the reflection. It is a good idea to remind the supervisee how much time she has left. For example, if 20 minutes has been negotiated, you might say, after 15 minutes, we have 5 minutes left for this issue. Often this can help move things on, whereas waiting until the 20 minutes are up may take the supervisee by surprise and leave her dissatisfied. If more time is needed to complete the reflection, this can always be renegotiated. For example, the supervisor might say 'We do not quite seem to have got to the bottom of this. What do you want to do?' It is then up to the supervisee to decide whether she wants to carry on or whether it would be more beneficial to her to move on to the next issue.

Clarity regarding topic

Clarity regarding the topic is related to the use of time. However, it may not be enough to be told by the supervisee 'Well I should like to talk about two of my clients, I think I will need about 30 minutes for the first one and 15 for the second.' It is a good start, but I want to know about the clients that the supervisee wants to look at. Often the supervisee will begin to talk in order to provide the supervisor with some of the 'facts'. This is useful because without knowing what happened, and a bit of context, we would be working in the dark. However, there can be a tendency for the supervisee to talk and talk at this point, swamping the supervisor with detail. Now, on the one hand, this does serve the supportive function of supervision, in that it can be a good way to off-load. However, unless the supervisee said that all she wants from bringing the issue is to off-load, spending too much time on 'the story' may not leave much time for any reflection. Clearly this is not a good use of time.

Experienced supervisees often come to supervision prepared. They have thought about what to bring, what they want from the session and 'how to get it'. In other words, they have learnt how to 'cut to the chase' as it were, giving a synopsis of the situation, which involves knowing what is important and what is peripheral. Supervisors can do a great deal to foster this skill by demonstrating it. The skill of summarising helps here. For example, after the supervisee has talked for 10 minutes about a complicated situation, the supervisor might say, 'So what you seem to be saying is that...' (here the supervisor gives a synopsis of what she has heard). It can also be helpful to ask questions such as: Could you say, in three sentences, what the main issue is? Or, what single word would describe this? Or, what image comes to mind when you think of this? By being asked questions like this the supervisee is helped to focus on what is most significant for her.

Identifying the 'what': what is the supervision question?

This involves helping supervisees to focus on what they want from the session. What is it they are not clear on? What do they want to know? What outcome do they want from the session? In other words, what is their goal?

Supervisees may know what the overall question is, but need to feel safe enough to bring it out into the open. There are various reasons for this. They may fear being judged, be embarrassed or feel emotionally wobbly; perhaps the issue is hitting a sensitive spot. Good listening skills are therefore essential, both to what is being said, but also to what is not being said but may be lurking just below the surface. When I am training novice supervisors, they often say things like 'I know that there is something there, I have a feeling that I am missing something, but I do not know what it is.' This is a good starting point. If that is how you feel, why not share that with the supervisee? This skill is called 'thinking aloud'. For example, you might say: 'I have a feeling that there is something else going on, but I am not sure what it is; what do you think?' This then gives the supervisee a chance to say what it is they really want – it is giving them permission as it were. So, it is a good idea to enlist the supervisee in the identification of the supervision question. Also, indicating that you look below the surface helps supervisees to engage in a deeper reflection and to develop the self-supervision skills that will facilitate their growth and development. Supervision carried out in this way is treating the supervisee like a co-investigator, and is therefore unlikely to create dependency.

Even when supervisees are clear on what they want to bring, the reason for it is not always obvious. The example in the previous chapter is a case in point. Sonia was clear on the two cases she wanted to talk about and how much time was needed for this. However, when she started to talk it was not immediately clear what the issue was. All she was aware of was a feeling of discomfort, but she did not really say what she wanted from the session. This became apparent when I asked her questions such as: What is it about this that concerns you? This helped Sonia to say that it had something to do with imposing the values of society on people. She then unpacked the situation a bit further so that I had a sense of what had happened. However, we still had not really established what outcome she would like, so I asked, 'What is it you would like to achieve as a result of talking about it?' This helped her to say that she wanted to unravel things a bit, but we still needed to focus in some more. That is why I decided to summarise her feelings: 'So are you saying that ... that you are feeling somewhat uncomfortable with the position that you are in the ... although it was necessary and nothing else could have been done, at the same time it feels heavy-handed. I don't know, is that what you are saying? Is that what you want to look at today?' I made my summary tentative, in order to give Sonia the opportunity to correct me if I had it wrong, or had misunderstood something. I guessed that somewhere in what she had been saying there was the focus, which is why I decided to go for it and ask her outright. This then helped us to move on to Step 2 and focus deeper on her feelings about the situation.

Overt and covert questions

A supervisee may come to a session saying 'I am not sure what is going on with ... and I don't know why.' Or, 'I have a sense that I am missing something, it is at the edge of my consciousness, but somehow I seem unable to access it.' The overt question is 'Help me get clarity and find out what is happening.' However, there may also be a more covert question: 'Am I doing all right?' or, 'If I did not do all right, what was it that got in the way and how can I prevent it happening again?' or, 'How can I do things differently, at the moment I seem to be at a loss.' It is good to develop the habit of listening to what is being asked beyond the overt questions, which involves listening to what is said as well as to what is not said. The supervisee may or may not be consciously aware what the covert question is, so it is up to the supervisor to develop that 'sixth sense' which will become easier as the relationship develops and the people concerned get to know each other.

Qualities

As discussed in the section on developing a working agreement in Chapter 2, the ability to develop a relationship with someone is crucial. Although this ability is important for both parties, I think the onus is on the supervisor. A quality of openness is very helpful, by which I mean being yourself and not pretending to be more or less experienced or knowledgeable than you are. This is something I learnt through experience. When I was first placed in a position of having to provide clinical supervision I, like so many others in my position, had not received any training at all. The only type of supervision I had received myself had been client-centred, so I modelled myself my own style on that experience. When it was time to review, the supervisee said, 'Yes, I do find you a good role model in that you really demonstrate the person-centred approach and the qualities associated with it. And yet ... I would like more of "you".' When we discussed this further the supervisee said that my non-directive style was not what she wanted. In a way she felt that I was holding out on her and denying her the benefit of my knowledge and experience. I on my part felt both flattered and disappointed. I felt flattered to be credited with potentially useful knowledge and experience, but I felt disappointed with myself for not having provided her with what she needed. I realised that it was time to look into supervision deeper, which led to training courses and the development of a wider range of responses and interventions. My experience is another example of the difference between counselling and supervision and an indication of the necessity (for client-centred practitioners at any rate) to develop a more authoritative style of working (Page & Wosket 2001:97).

Comfortable with 'not knowing'

When the supervision relationship is new, neither of us really knows how a session will feel, or how the other person will react to what we say or do. Whether I am in the role of supervisor or supervisee I find it helpful to pretend to myself that every session is a first session and that I have no idea what is going to happen. In a way this is always correct, as we can never know that. Preparing by giving myself a few minutes of quiet time before a session also helps with this attitude. As a supervisor, an attitude of 'not knowing' means that I cannot take anything for granted and really have to focus on the supervisee and what she is bringing (Moore 1995:57).

Principles of 'not knowing'

An important principle of a 'not knowing' attitude is to start from where the supervisee is; this means that you have to find out. Even if I feel that I have had a fairly thorough introductory chat with a supervisee, I do not think that I can then assume that I know exactly where they are in their experience or development. Basically I find that people have a unique talent for being surprising. For example, students or trainees may have more insight than you expect. There can be a great deal of variation between people who appear to be at the same stage of training. It is therefore not helpful to assume that we already know what goes on between a practitioner and another person. In any case, we were not there, so in a real sense we can never know. All we can do is to use our skills to get a sense of the encounter, so that we can help the supervisee reflect on what is needed.

Also, even if we have worked with a supervisee for a while, to assume that we know does not allow for the possibility of that person's continuous growth and development. Trainees are not the only people who can be surprising, as very experienced people may have unexpected gaps in their experience or blind spots that they may not themselves be aware of. So, as a supervisee it is good to let your supervisor know you and your level of development. This means not only a sharing of what you are good at, but also of what is lacking, what you find difficult and what needs further developing. This may be uncomfortable, but if it is not done it may take a while before both of you really get into the process and you may not get the supervision that you need. So, the better the relationship, the easier people will find it to be honest and open in talking about difficult material. Clearly it is not reasonable to expect this to happen from day one; relationships need time to develop but, as in any other relationship, both parties must be willing.

Attitude of respectful curiosity: supervision as enquiry

Corbett quotes TS Elliot as saying 'If we want to discover something we must approach it by way of not knowing, not by way of already knowing' (Corbett in Kugler 1995:74). It is therefore good to retain an attitude of respectful curiosity, and to see a supervision session as an enquiry or research, something to find out about. I believe that an attitude of not knowing and respectful curiosity is also the one to adopt with clients. After all, no matter how experienced we are, and how many people we have met who appeared to have the same kind of problem, we simply cannot know, without listening to them, what the experience is like for this particular person.

A trainee counsellor told me how he felt let down by his supervisor, despite seeing her for an hour every week. The trainee had been working with a rather borderline client for more than a year, when things became difficult. Despite saying this in supervision he felt that the difficulties were not really engaged with and ultimately the client left prematurely. The counsellor felt that he had let down his client as he had been let down by his supervisor. When I asked what the problem was the counsellor said that he had never felt safe enough in the supervision to say how he really felt. He had felt judged rather than held and was therefore unable to hold the client when things became difficult. An attitude of respectful enquiry might have helped him. If the supervisor had been able to be with the counsellor in a warm, yet enquiring way, the client in turn might have felt safe enough to stay.

For example, the supervisor might have role-modelled how to be with the client by saying 'So what is happening for you is "X"? What is happening for me is "Y". What are we going to do about that?' This would have created a space for true dialogue and enquiry. There would no longer have been a need for the counsellor to hide what was going on.

Skills

The skills of active listening, questioning, summarising and focusing are crucial to Step 1 as well as to the other two sections of the supervision process. They are also the cause of people sometimes getting confused regarding the difference between counselling and supervision. This is because these skills are also sometimes known as counselling skills. However, just because activities require similar skills that does not mean that the activities themselves are the same. For example, both a politician and a car salesman need the ability to make people enthusiastic about what they tell them, they need to be able to persuade. Clearly it would be incorrect to say that the man who sells you your new car is doing exactly the same thing as a government minister. Yes, there are some skills that are similar, it may even be the case that some of these skills are transferable between the two activities, but that is where it ends. Similarly with counselling and supervision. In counselling the 'basic' active listening, focusing and questioning skills are used to help the person explore their inner world. In supervision, however, the focus is on the practitioner's work, the situations they encounter and the clients they work with. The helping professions also involve a 'therapeutic use of self', which requires a certain level of self-awareness. Indeed such self-awareness is intimately bound up with the development of the 'internal supervisor'. If it becomes clear that there is something in the supervisee's inner world that stands in the way of working effectively, it is the supervisor's job to point this out and to suggest alternative ways, such as individual counselling, to deal with this.

Active listening

Active listening means not only hearing what the other person is saying, it also involves letting the other person know that you have heard and understood them, to encourage the other person to go on talking. This is done by responding both verbally and non-verbally. Non-verbal responses may take the form of nodding or encouragers such as hmm, uhm. Verbal response may be simple encouragers, such as 'go on' or 'tell me more', or they may take the form of reflection or paraphrase. A paraphrase is basically saying back to the person what they have just said in a slightly different way. Reflection may be of fact or of feeling. Reflection of fact basically says back to the person what they have just told you, using more or less the same words, whereas reflection of feeling picks up on the feeling with which something was expressed. (For a more in-depth explanation of active listening skills see van Ooijen 2000:83–87.)

Questioning

There is an art to questioning. As a general rule, only ask closed questions (which require a yes, no or specific answer) if you want to know something specific. If you want to encourage the supervisee to explore their thinking ask an open question, to which there is no specific answer. For example, 'What do you feel about the client?', or 'How did you see that?' (see van Ooijen 2000:110–113 for a more in-depth discussion).

Summarising

This is a very useful skill as it helps to consolidate material and put it in a nutshell as it were, after which the discussion can move on.

Focusing

This involves helping the supervisee, by focused questioning, to become clear on what exactly it is that concerns them. A focusing question can often be usefully asked after a summary. For example, a supervisor might say to a social work supervisee, 'So you feel that the situation has become very complicated over the past few weeks as there are a number of different agencies involved. You are charged with the task of coordination and action, but what is not clear to me is what in this situation you want to look at today.' As you can see, the focusing is done by means of a question, which leaves it up to the supervisee to become more specific. I feel that it is important to beware of focusing too narrowly too soon. This is because, once we select something for attention, inevitably something else will get ignored as there is only so much we can do at any one time. The supervisor needs to be aware of this, and try to avoid bias either by himself or by the supervisee being too selective in what to bring. I mentioned earlier that if supervisees feel unsafe or patronised they might become rather selective in what they bring to supervision. It is important to keep an eye out for this. If I notice that a supervisee never talks about certain aspects of her job I may ask about that when it feels appropriate. I may also wonder whether it is something I do that prevents her from doing so. Ultimately, though, supervision is for the supervisee, therefore it has to be conducted in a way that facilitates her to work well, and to grow and develop. Being cajoled into seeing and doing things in line with a supervisor's particular point of view is unlikely to do so.

Methods

The most helpful method, tool or technique in Step 1 is preparation.

Preparation by the supervisor

As a supervisor I like to prepare by having a brief period of quiet time so that I can centre myself. I find this helps me to get a sense of how I am feeling; the brief rest helps me regenerate and be better able to create the supervision space. Obviously, such a brief quiet time is equally useful for supervisees. After a 'mis/take' I now extend the getting a sense of how I am feeling before a supervision session to telephone calls. If I am feeling upset, very tired or pre-occupied, I let the answering machine take the message. A few years ago I had had an informal conversation with a prospective supervisee and we had agreed to start working together. Normally I would discuss my version of the working agreement; I then tend to give it to people to take away and think about. However, for reasons that are not relevant here this had not been done so that the supervisee was unaware of my 48-hour cancellation period. The day before I was due to see him again I was actually very angry about something totally unrelated to my work. This had the effect that when the prospective supervisee rang to say that he could not make it the next day I said, 'Well, I do have to charge.' Later I realised that I had made a mistake. In fact, I could not even send a bill as I had not yet found out who in his organisation was responsible for paying it. I was therefore not surprised when the person decided not to start working with me, in fact I never saw him again. Needless to say, I have learnt from the experience and will not make that particular mistake again.

Preparation by the supervisee – a reflective log

It is good to get into the habit of regular reflection and preparation before a supervision session, in order to start thinking about a desirable outcome or goal. I would encourage anyone working in the helping professions to keep a journal or reflective log. Over the years I have found such a log invaluable and a great help when it comes to producing a portfolio or file of evidence as is now required by so many of our accrediting organisations. How often you make an entry in such a log is up to you; however, I would suggest doing it at least weekly. If you can do it daily, so much the better; it need not be long, a few sentences will probably suffice. See if you can set some time aside each week, ideally at the same time, to reflect on the week and record everything that has stayed in your mind. Then, when it comes to your supervision, you can make a selection from your reflective log. It can be quite interesting to look at a log over a period of a few months, in order to see whether there are certain themes that keep popping up. If so, these are certainly useful to bring to supervision.

How to present the material

In order to make the most effective use of supervision it is good to learn the skills of organising the material you wish to bring and to learn to present it in a way that is concise and to the point. Once I had a supervisor who would shout 'enough' if I talked for more than 5 minutes. His view was that there is no need to know a great deal – what he wanted was the essence. Although I did not like it at the time, this was a good learning experience. It helped me reflect beforehand on what exactly the issue was and how I could present it clearly, accurately and concisely. It is a good habit to get into and a useful skill to learn, as it means that most of the supervision session can be spent on reflection, rather than on more and more detailed information – which is likely to confuse rather than clarify things. It can be helpful to ask yourself questions such as:

- What do I feel about this?
- What does it mean to me?
- When have I felt like this before?
- What was the issue then? (van Ooijen 2000:59)

Tools and techniques

Having said above that it is a good idea to prepare for supervision, from time to time I like to do something spontaneous. Sometimes preparation can be rather rational and not leave much space for the emotional or non-rational. However, clinical supervision aims to achieve a 'super' vision, which means a shift in that vision, a shift in our consciousness. The intention of supervision is for practitioners to increase their self-knowledge as well as their understanding of others, whether these others are clients, colleagues or managers. Ultimately supervision is about supporting us to develop safe and effective ways of working, either directly or indirectly. Our current society and the climate within which many of us work places great emphasis on research, evidence-based practice, standards and problem-solving. Although all this is necessary, there is a tendency to over-focus on our rational capabilities, which can have the effect of neglecting our non-rational, intuitive abilities. However, it is those non-rational capabilities that so often characterise the expert worker (Benner & Wrubel 1989). The expert often does not have to follow a problem-solving protocol, but will somehow 'know' what is the right thing to do. Creative methods are increasingly recognised as having something useful to offer in this area. Supervision requires us to reflect – on ourselves and how we work, on our clients and others that we come into contact with as part of our working day. But reflection is not easy. After having supervision for a while, people often say something like: 'I thought I used to reflect, that supervision held nothing new for me, but now I realise that was not true. The way in which I reflected in the past was actually rather superficial, and the reason for that was often that it was largely factual and rational.'

Creative methods, art, poetry, literature, visualisations, to name but a few, all aim to focus on our non-rational mind, on our emotional and intuitive abilities, which are so important in dealing with people. A selection of creative methods is outlined below. They are intended as an alternative method of topic selection and focusing on what is needed. They can also be used by the supervisee as a means of preparing for their supervision.

Speaking as an object

Here the supervisee is asked to think of their work area and then speak as the first object or person that comes to mind.

 EXAMPLE

I am the resuscitation trolley. I am very important really, but people tend to only remember me when I am wanted suddenly. I am not always replenished properly as I should be. I should be cleaned and checked regularly, but this does not happen, no-one seems to be responsible for me. Sometimes people borrow things from me and do not put them back, so next time I am needed, things are missing and people get very angry. This makes me feel bad because it is not my fault yet I feel guilty. I also feel angry; they should look after me properly and maintain me better, so that I can do my work.

This example clearly demonstrates how the supervisee felt about her work. She was surprised at the strength of her feelings, as she had previously said that things were fine and that there were no problems. It is an example of how creative methods can go below the defences I discussed earlier. The supervisor was then able to help her clarify her thoughts and feelings further, which led to a useful discussion of what she could do to change things.

Poetry

Give the supervisee a line and then give her 3 minutes to write a poem, without thinking about it too much, or worry about whether or not it rhymes. Here is an example from a counsellor who was given the line 'I have a client who ...':

I have a client who
Is slowly driving me mad
I've seen her for a long, long time
But we're not getting anywhere
Is it me or is it her
What do I want to happen
Should I challenge
Or just be there
Am I doing all right
What is so different
I ask myself
She seems happy enough
Am I afraid of
What's underneath
Am I avoiding
What?

Another useful first sentence may be: 'The last time I was working, someone said to me ...' Here is an example from a physiotherapist:

The last time I was working
someone said to me
I felt really touched
just now, it was
a moving experience.
Thank you, I said
and resisted the urge
to minimise her words
and reflect them away.
There was no need
It was her experience
To learning, to growing

To the space and the time
To care
And it felt good
To leave it – there.

This is a good example of how supervision is also about celebrating positive experiences and to help consolidate them, so that we can feel good about them. Doing this helps to develop people's confidence to own their own good practice, and to continue practising in that way. Here is another example, this time from a worker in a hospice:

It was difficult to feel the pain
to tolerate just staying there
I saw in her eyes
That she sensed my confusion
So I held her hand.

I had nothing more to offer
Than just being me
Although I wanted
To run away …
I relaxed.

And suddenly I knew
I did not have to do
Anything … beyond
Just to be there … with her.

Again, this was a positive experience, but it was also difficult. The supervisee felt ambivalent about her experience. She knew that the patient sensed her discomfort and did not know how to deal with that. So she needed to be held herself, in supervision, so that she could hold the patient. In other words, she needed support to help her tolerate the pain of another human being, which we can only do if we receive help ourselves. But also she needed help to see that she was in fact simply being herself. The patient sensed her discomfort, but at the same time also knew that despite that discomfort she stayed there with the patient. She was real, herself, just another human being and that was just what was needed.

The use of music

Play a piece of music; ask people to close their eyes and adopt a comfortable position so they can really relax. Then say the following:

Listen to the music, whilst mindful of your work. Perhaps you find yourself thinking of a particular client or situation ... whatever it is that comes to mind ... keep it within your consciousness. Notice, without judging what happens ... what images, memories, words or fragments of conversations come into your awareness. Resist the temptation to dwell on anything, just continue listening and noticing.

Say this slowly, pausing regularly to give people a chance to get into the visualisation. Then bring them back by saying:

Bring yourself back now to where you are, feel the touch of your clothes on your skin, the weight of your body on the chair (or the floor), and the air against your face. In a few moments I will count to three and on the count of three you may open your eyes. One ... two ... three.

Rapid writing

Here you give your supervisee the following instructions: 'Think of a work situation or a client. Now write for 3 minutes without thinking about it, just write, do not let your pen lift from the paper.' Or you could ask the supervisee to write: 'When I was in work the other day, someone said to me ...' and then to continue writing.

Alternatively, you could ask people to draw or paint whatever comes to mind. I find that, whenever I use methods like this, people are often surprised at what surfaces. 'I thought I had dealt with that issue,' they may say, 'but I realise now that I haven't.'

 EXAMPLE

A senior social worker drew a tightrope with three people. One was dancing on one end, barely touching the rope, one was almost falling off at the other end. In the middle he had drawn himself, trying to hold the balance. This graphic portrayal of a difficult situation within the team provided a very clear focus for the supervision session. It was interesting as consciously the supervisee thought that he was handling the situation well. In other words, he had not let himself be sufficiently aware that there was a problem that needed to be looked at.

A note of caution

Before using creative methods it is wise to check out how the supervisee feels about the idea, as there are people who just do not like using them. If this were the case, I would not push it, as that is likely to be counter-productive.

CONCLUSION

In summary, the focus of the supervision session is determined by asking the supervisee what they want to bring, what their objective is in doing so, what they want to achieve as a result and what the real issue appears to be. In general, it is good to ask supervisees to come prepared, although from time to time it can be useful to make use of creative methods within the session.

Step 1 may be summarised as follows:

- How many clients/issues do you want to bring today?
- How much time do you think you need for each?
- What do you want to achieve as a result?
- How do you want to feel when we finish talking about it?

In the next chapter I discuss how the work that was begun in Step 1 can be continued and further developed in Step 2.

Questions for further reflection

- How do you currently view mistakes – either your own or those made by your supervisee?

- Have you experienced problems in a supervisory relationship? If so, what happened? How would you deal with it if it happened again?

- Which of the above skills, tools and techniques might you wish to incorporate in your practice?

- What are your reasons for this choice?

5

Reflecting in supervision: working with the 'how' section

Supervision ... must start with reflecting on the concrete experience and try to make sense of this in a way that allows the experience to challenge one's own way of seeing and thinking about the world. (Hawkins & Shohet 2000:177)

In this chapter I discuss what to do once the focus and desired outcomes of a session have been agreed. The skills, qualities and tasks associated with Step 2 are given detailed attention, as well as what to do when things go wrong.

 EXAMPLE: STOP, LOOK AND LISTEN

Lynn, a counsellor in private practice, was in full flow. She had told me that she felt stuck in working with John, a man in his forties, and wanted to look at why this was, so that she could do something about it. She talked and talked and talked. I tried to interrupt her a few times, but she did not seem to hear me. I was beginning to get a headache, as I felt I was being given too much information in one go, I just could not take it in. In the end I said, 'STOP.' She stopped, startled. 'Lynn,' I said, 'I must tell you what is happening for me. I feel that you are keeping me out, there is so much that you are telling me, it feels quite overwhelming, but I am not being given a chance to say or do anything. So how can we do anything useful?' At first Lynn looked a bit annoyed, then she burst out laughing. 'Oh dear, I see what you are doing. I am being my client, aren't I.' 'Aha,' I said, 'but now you are back, so let us look at this.'

STARTING STEP 2

Whatever is decided in Step 1 will determine the focus and process of Step 2. All too often people simply dive in and start reflecting on aspects of what the supervisee brings or even giving advice, without knowing whether that is what is wanted. In the above example I knew what it was that Lynn wanted – to know what was causing the stuckness between her and her client. She then proceeded to behave in exactly the same way as her client, but without knowing that she was doing it. So, although she did not realise it, she was doing exactly what needed to be done in order to work with what she had brought. (This phenomenon is called parallel process and will be discussed later.) What I mean to make clear by this example is that in Step 2 we can give ourselves the freedom to reflect in whatever way is needed. Reflection, if it is done well, involves the left brain as well as the right brain, the rational and the non-rational, thinking and feeling, as well as intuition, hunches and physical sensations. In other words, reflection is not just a straightforward logical process, it can also involve the more murky aspects of our experience. As the above example shows, it can help us to become aware of what is below the surface.

THE SKILLS, QUALITIES AND TASKS OF STEP 2

Table 5.1 sets out the tasks to be accomplished at Step 2, as well as helpful skills and qualities. The qualities and skills listed are those most pertinent to this particular step, but this does not mean that they are not relevant to the other two steps. For example, I see self-awareness on the part of the supervisor as particularly relevant to the 'how' step, because it is here that the supervisee is helped to engage in a deeper reflection and thus develop a greater self-awareness. If we have not gone down that self-awareness road ourselves we are unlikely to be able to help the supervisee very far along the way. In a way a supervisor is a guide on the road of reflection and, like any guide, we can only go as far as we have been before or we may get lost.

Table 5.1   Step 2: facilitating reflection on the 'how'

	Supervisor	Supervisee

Tasks	Create a reflective space
	Facilitate integration of theory and practice
	Help supervisees feel safe and supported
	Co-creation of meaning with the
	   supervisee
		Develop the internal
		   supervisor
		Further develop
		   self-awareness
		Ensuring best
		   practice

Qualities,
  skills and
  methods
	Self-awareness
	Honesty
	Able to tolerate not knowing
	Self-supervision
	Helicopter skills
	Observe supervisee's reactions and
	   reflecting back when appropriate
	Sensitive questioning
	Reflection of difficult material
	Constructive criticism
	Supportive challenge
	Overcoming stuckness
	Knowing what to do when things go wrong
	Appropriate use of models
	Working with the non-rational
	Using creative methods – designed to tap
	   those areas that 'just talking' does not
	   reach
		Self-awareness
		Honesty
		Able to tolerate not
		   knowing
		Self-supervision

HOLDING THE BOUNDARY

The supervisor needs to help supervisees feel safe and supported by holding the boundary between supervision and counselling. Although supervision is not counselling or therapy, it can be therapeutic. As discussed in Chapter 2, it is important not to stray into counselling, as not only may this cause the supervisee to feel unsafe, it may also be in breach of the working agreement. However, sometimes what is happening in the practitioner's personal life may be relevant. Gilbert and Evans give a good example of how it is possible to engage with a supervisee's personal feelings without straying into counselling or therapy, in order to illuminate what is going on in their relationship with a client (Gilbert & Evans 2000:29–34). In the example, the supervisee is helped to see how his reactions to a client are rooted in his personal history. This insight is then used to throw further light on his work with the client, but at no time is his personal background submitted to any further scrutiny. Of course, after such an insight the supervisee may well decide to discuss the issue further with a counsellor, a friend or a family member, but that is entirely up to the supervisee and outside the remit of supervision. If, on the other hand, it would seem that the personal material is getting in the way of the practitioner being able to work effectively, it would be good for the supervisor to check with the supervisee that they have somewhere where they can discuss it further. So, although in therapy and counselling the focus is on the personal and in supervision on the work, if supervision is practised optimally we can potentially learn much about ourselves in supervision. And whatever we learn about ourselves in therapy or supervision can of course be fruitfully used in our work. Increased self-awareness can help us to understand our clients better. It can also aid us in engaging more openly in supervision. As we gain more self-awareness and feel safe within the working alliance, we can, hopefully, gradually let go of some of our defences and become more open and honest about who we are and how we work.

INTEGRATING THEORY AND PRACTICE

In Step 2 the supervisee is helped to look deeper into the 'what' that was chosen in Step 1, with the aim to discover more about 'how' things happened and what reasons there might be for this (Steel 2002). It is not sufficient just to gain experience without also reflecting on what we experience in order to learn from it. Most of us can probably think of people who, despite having been around in their profession for a long time, have not been in the habit of reflecting on that experience. As a result they do not appear to have learnt a great deal and may seem quite rigid in their approach to their work. They seem to do things out of habit, and when challenged will say this is because 'We have always done it this way.' By definition, reflection on experience implies a willingness to learn, openness to discovering new knowledge and perhaps seeing things in a different way. For some of us this may seem threatening as it may challenge us to let go of cherished beliefs and attitudes. However, facilitated reflection is an excellent aid in helping us move along the developmental path from novice to expert, for which integration of experience and theory is crucial.

Theory and practice cannot exist without each other. Although it is interesting to know why something happens, without relevant experience we will not know what to do. For example, a student nurse may have learnt what causes a stroke or a heart attack; she may even have a fairly good knowledge of what happens in the body physiologically. However, this general knowledge will not help her when faced with a particular patient who is having a heart attack in front of her. Even being told what to do is not sufficient; what she needs is experience. Whereas theoretical knowledge is necessarily at the level of the general – 'This is what happens when someone has a heart attack' – experience is always at the level of the particular. 'What is happening with this person, here and now and what do I need to do that is helpful' are questions that the student nurse needs to have answers to if she is to develop into a competent professional. An expert combines general knowledge with the experience of lots of particular instances. She is able to integrate the two because she has reflected on what happened with particular people and related that back to theoretical knowledge. Her experience has become grounded in theory and the theory has become grounded in her experience. Facilitation of this process is part of the educative function of supervision. In order to learn from our experience we need the time and space to think about it, in order to make sense of it, so that we can be more effective next time we encounter a similar situation.

The qualities of self-awareness, honesty and the ability to tolerate not knowing what is going on are important to cultivate for supervisor and supervisee alike. Before we can make sense of anything, we need to give it time and resist the temptation to jump to premature conclusions. To help us make sense of why things happen we need to start with what happens. We can facilitate this process by saying something like 'What exactly happened, let's look at this' and then help the supervisee to look at it from all angles. This involves not only the observable facts of the situation, but also what thoughts, feelings and sensations the supervisee had at the time – and what she is experiencing now that she is talking about it. It is also helpful to try to get a sense of how the client or other relevant people may be experiencing things.

CREATING THE SPACE FOR REFLECTION

When I go on holiday I like to be unrushed and to give myself time and space to enjoy, reflect, eat well, read good books, walk, swim and enjoy just being. In a way, creating the supervision space is a bit like encouraging the supervisee to 'hold on to that holiday feeling'. Sometimes, when a supervisee feels very stressed, or wants to rush ahead and give me more and more details about something, I may ask: 'What do you like to do on holiday?' and then, 'How can you be more like that here (or in your work)?'

Creating the space for reflection is the most important task at Step 2. It is tremendously helpful to have a supervisor who really wants to know about you and your work. As a supervisee I want my supervisor to listen with complete attention, to be interested in my thoughts, feelings, hunches, uncertainties and general musings. I also want them to share with me their reactions to the material I bring as well as pertinent comments on 'how' I bring it. For example, do I seem irritable, anxious, blasé, pleased, stressed or angry? In other words, I want them to work with the there and then (my work) as well as the here and now (me talking about my work with my supervisor).

Reflection on our thoughts, feelings and actions is not a new idea. The Greek philosopher Socrates was well known for his dialogues, which could be seen as facilitated reflection. After engaging in such a dialogue with Socrates people tended to have a different view of things – something had opened up, a shift had taken place, making room for a more creative way of thinking. Socrates did this by allowing plenty of space for the reflection and by challenging cherished beliefs, assumptions or ways of thinking.

Allowing plenty of space for reflection is crucial to the success of the supervision. I often find myself saying to people 'Do less and you will probably achieve a lot more.' Don't be too anxious to be seen to know all the answers; that really is an impossible burden to create for yourself. Supervision is about creating a space in which both parties really let themselves engage with the material, to enable a greater clarity to emerge.

Page and Wosket see the space section of their Cyclical Model, which was discussed in Chapter 1, as the 'heart' of the supervision process (Page & Wosket 2001:103). Oh, I hear you say, I need to create a space for reflection and also challenge the supervisee when appropriate. But how do I get them to reflect and what should they be reflecting on? It is at this point that Hawkins and Shohet's Seven-Eyed Model comes into its own as it offers a number of different ways of looking at things (Hawkins & Shohet 2000:67–87).

Creating a reflective space

According to Hawkins and Shohet, any issue, situation or practitioner–client relationship can be looked at from seven different angles, called 'eyes', 'modes' or 'foci':

1. What actually happened (the facts)?
2. What did the practitioner actually do – what strategies did he employ, what tools did he use?
3. What is the relationship like between the practitioner and the other person?
4. What is going on inside the practitioner – both when he is with the client and when he thinks or talks about them?
5. What is happening in the relationship between the supervisor and the supervisee?
6. What is going on inside the supervisor?
7. What is the context within which the work as well as the supervision takes place? (Hawkins & Shohet 2000:67–87)

Modes 1–3 focus on what happened 'out there' – Hawkins and Shohet call this the Therapy Matrix – whereas in modes 4–6 the focus is on what is happening in the supervision session itself (the Supervision Matrix). However, the purpose of the reflection in the Supervision Matrix is to throw light on whatever it is that the supervisee has brought.

The seven different foci are all legitimate areas for reflection in Step 2, but which of them are chosen will depend on the developmental level of the supervisee, the professional context and the experience, the preference of the supervisor and what feels appropriate at the time. According to Hawkins and Shohet there is a more or less linear relationship between the appropriateness of the focus (from 1 to 6) and the developmental level of the worker. With inexperienced workers, for example, it is probably a good idea to spend time on finding out what happened as well as on what they actually did. Also those in the more factually (non-mental health) oriented professions such as general nursing may feel that finding out what happened and what was done is an important part of supervision. Counsellors and others whose main job involves working with people's mental well-being will find it beneficial to focus on their relationships with clients as well as on their own internal experience. Working with the supervisory relationship as well as with the supervisor's own experience is likely to be helpful, irrespective of the professional or theoretical orientation of the worker. However, in my experience, unless people are already interested in a psychodynamic way of working they may need to experience the effectiveness of this first before they are convinced that this is a useful thing to do. I will discuss this further in the next chapter under the heading 'working with the non-rational'.

THE PRESSURE TO BE EFFICIENT

Reflection has its own rhythm, so there is value in working slowly. However, this is against our current climate of wanting instant answers and immediate solutions. Sometimes people say that with trainees and inexperienced practitioners there is no time for a reflective space as their supervisees have so much to learn. Helping the supervisee to reflect on their experience and come up with helpful strategies is seen as an inefficient use of time as it is far quicker simply to tell them what to do. If you work in a highly pressured environment where time is regarded as a scarce commodity, this may seem a reasonable point of view. But my answer is that it does not work, not in the long run anyway. Whereas, initially, supervisees may be pleased to be given an answer to a problem they may have, others are likely to be frustrated as they would prefer to be helped to come up with their own solutions. They may well have a few ideas already and would welcome the opportunity to discuss them. I would argue that it is far more effective to help people 'own' their strategies and solutions. Not only does this make it more likely that they will carry them out, they are also likely to do them more effectively as they are already in agreement. Doing what someone else tells you to do may not feel quite right or a bit uncomfortable and may cause the strategy to be less effective.

So, I am holding up a torch here for plenty of reflective space in Step 2, irrespective of the developmental level of the supervisee. However, 'what' we expect a supervisee to reflect on, become aware of and think about must, of course, be in line with where they are in their own development. Clearly it would be unreasonable to expect a novice practitioner to function at the level of an expert.

Is developmental supervision different?

It could be argued that regarding supervision as either serving a developmental or a consultative function is a matter of differing emphasis rather than emphatic difference. It would seem uncontroversial to say that to help a student or practitioner to develop their own insight and solution is always a good idea and should not in itself be dependent on their stage of development. Facilitating a student to develop their capacity for thinking, reflection and problem solving is in fact fundamental to good teaching, and as argued above, crucial in helping them to integrate theory and practice. It can be really annoying and demotivating to be 'told' too much, without having had the opportunity to get there for yourself.

 EXAMPLE

Brian, an experienced occupational therapist, had recently moved to another department, which meant working with a different client group than he was used to. Although he had much to learn about this new area, he also felt that a great deal of his existing knowledge and experience was transferable, but that his new supervisor, Sally, did not recognise that. He role-played a typical scenario:

Supervisee: Blah, blah, blah (talking about a client).

Supervisor: Perhaps … is happening, you could try ….

Supervisee: *Thinks* – no, she is on the wrong track, anyway I have already considered that. *Says* – uhm, well, I thought of that but I don't think that is the case here actually.

Supervisor: Have you checked it out. What I think is going on is … (reiterates what she had said already in a slightly different way).

Supervisee: *Thinks* – oh dear, she's off again, now I will have to sit through another 5 minutes of her going on. Perhaps it is easier just to let her talk. *After 5 minutes* – yes, interesting, maybe. *Has given up; thinks* – I must change my supervisor, this is not getting anywhere but I do feel that I need help, what a pain.

 THINKING POINT

What is going on here do you think?

The supervisor is giving her opinions as well as suggested strategies before the supervisee has been facilitated to reflect on the situation. This is never a good idea as even in a training situation advice or information given too early is demotivating. Often this is the result of the supervisor's enthusiasm and eagerness to do the best by the supervisee. Sometimes, though, it may be serving the needs of the supervisor to be seen as all knowledgeable or powerful. Or it may be that the supervisor is insecure and wants to keep the sessions under her control as much as possible. Perhaps she feels that she cannot cope, or that her lack of knowledge or experience could be exposed if she asks the supervisee to do a lot of reflecting. Most of the time this fear is not warranted. It tends to be the really dedicated people who may feel inadequate, but they often know much more than they give themselves credit for. In any case, supervision is not about knowing all the answers, it is about allowing plenty of space to reflect on an issue. This means the ability not to be unnerved by not knowing what is going on, to refrain from rushing into premature clarity and to help both of you to trust that, given sufficient attention, answers will emerge.

The above situation was eventually resolved when Brian confronted Sally and told her that he wanted to leave as he did not feel valued or supported. Sally was surprised and a bit shocked at her own lack of awareness. Her openness about her own reaction reassured Brian and the two had a (belated) exchange about the supervision itself and how they were going to continue working together. Brian's example demonstrates how Step 2 can only be effective if the groundwork has been laid at Step 1.

DEVELOPMENT OF THE INTERNAL SUPERVISOR

Being facilitated to integrate theory and practice will go a long way towards the development of the internal supervisor. This is not the same as thinking 'What would my supervisor do if they were me?' – that would be an internalised supervisor. When new to a profession, having an internalised supervisor is not a bad idea. However, no-one wants lots of clones, because as human beings we have a duty to become as fully ourselves as we can be. This means that we need to develop an internal sense of how we work and why we work, something we can consult with when necessary. This self-supervision is probably close to the idea of 'reflection in action'; it means that we reflect on what is happening, while it is happening, in order to be as effective as we can be.

CO-CREATION OF MEANING

Practising supervision in a respectful way will go a long way towards helping people to feel safe and supported. If you create a climate in which it is safe to say anything, without fear of being judged or told off, your supervisees are likely to make good use of the space you offer (Fig. 5.1). For example, a supervisee may say 'I really need to off-load about this client because they are driving me mad.'

Consider the following supervisory responses:

1. That is no way to talk about a client, they come to you for support, not criticism.
2. You clearly still have a lot to learn about warmth, empathy and being non-judgemental.
3. Oh, Mrs J, yes, she is difficult isn't she. I'd prefer you to talk about someone else as I feel just as irritated as you. You just have drawn the short straw I'm afraid.
4. Oh yes, some clients are like that aren't they. I had a client last week who ... (proceeds to tell the story).
5. Tell me about her ... let's explore what is going on.

Which responses would make you feel safe and supported? No prizes for the right answer here! Although two of the five answers seem supportive, only the last response is likely to be helpful. There is no judging, of either the supervisee or the client – just an expression of interest, and a willingness to explore the situation and reflect upon it. Whereas responses 3 and 4 may help the supervisee to feel temporarily supported, only response 5 shines a torch on the issue and is therefore likely to help achieve that 'super' vision.

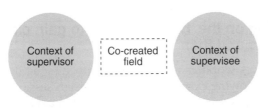

Figure 5.1   Co-creation of a safe space.

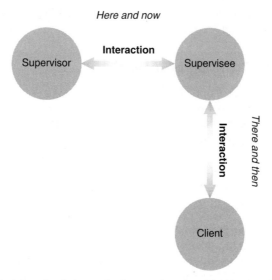

Here and now

Figure 5.2   Interaction between the 'here and now' and the 'there and then'.

When supervisor and supervisee reflect together, what emerges is co-created. Page & Wosket (2001:107) use the term 'reflective alliance' for this way of working. I really like this term as it encompasses the collaborative nature of supervision. In a supervisory alliance both supervisor and supervisee reflect on what might be going on, either out there (the supervisee's work) or in here (the supervision situation).

As is clear from the Seven-Eyed Model, at any one time we have a choice whether to focus on what happened 'out there' or on what is happening 'here and now' (see Fig. 5.2). Good supervision usually involves a smooth movement between these two main areas.

Focusing on the 'here and now' to gain clarity on the 'there and then'

This involves working with what is happening as it is happening. The following extract from a supervision session between a community psychiatric nurse (CPN) and his supervisor illustrates how this can work.

EXAMPLE

CPN: I just don't seem to be able to get through to this client.
                I feel we're just going through the motions.

Supervisor: Have the two of you talked about that?

CPN: Not as such. I just keep thinking of different angles
                to use.

Supervisor: Just now, when you were talking, I found myself
                thinking, I must think up some really good strategies
                that can be used. I wonder if she has tried x, y and z.
                I feel a real pull to help you sort it out.

CPN: That is just how I feel. The previous worker did not get
                anywhere, so I felt determined to be more successful.

Supervisor: And you don't feel that any of your strategies are
                working?

CPN: No, not really. Whatever I think of just seems to
                evaporate.

Supervisor: So anything I suggest might suffer the same fate
                I suppose.

CPN: Yes, and that would be really scary as then what would
                I do?

Supervisor: I find myself wondering how it feels to be talking like this?

CPN: Good, actually. I feel less desperate to find a solution or
                yet another technique to try. I don't really understand
                why as I still don't know what to do, but somehow
                finding yet another technique or strategy does not
                seem relevant anymore.

Supervisor: That is interesting, can you say a bit more?

CPN: Well, you know that last time you said that you like
                to be up-front with people? And just now you, I suppose
                you were very up-front with me. I'd like to do that
                with my client, to talk about what has been going on.

Supervisor: Can you say more?

CPN: Well, they would be more involved. I guess it would
                show more respect, less having things done to them.
                I could discuss with Mark how I am feeling and give him
                the opportunity to tell me how he feels that we are
                getting on. Perhaps I have been focusing on doing
                things to him rather than with him.

Supervisor: Hmm, that sounds like an important insight. Would you
                like us to try it out? What if I am the client, and you are
                yourself?

CPN: Yes, that is a good idea.

And so on.

The co-creation of meaning can feel like a mysterious process. A
supervisee may bring a client with a very distressing story and my
initial reaction may be, 'Help, what am I supposed to do here – and
she's coming to me for help?' It is likely that this is counter-transference (see next chapter) and that I am picking up how the supervisee
and indeed the client may be feeling. I have found time and again
that if I trust the co-creation and give it plenty of time, during which
we reflect and sit with it, meaning will somehow emerge.

Being up-front

In the 'here and now' focus we meet the other person where they
are, which means that we can be up-front about what we are experiencing at the time. In the above example the supervisor shared
her experience of the here and now, which facilitated the supervisee to realise what was going on for him in relation to his client.

BALANCING AWARENESS

*Effective supervision involves a delicate balance of
awareness and entails the capacity both to be in our
own experience, appreciate that of the other and stand
back in order to reflect on the interaction between the
two ...* (Gilbert & Evans 2000:21)

From the quote it is clear that Gilbert and Evans see supervisors as
constantly checking back with themselves and practising self-
supervision as they go along. For me that means that I listen to the

supervisee and then check in with myself for the effect it has on me. What do I catch myself thinking, what do I feel, do I have any sensation in my body that was not there previously? Then I move my focus back onto the supervisee and notice 'how' they talk, their tone of voice, facial expression and body language; then I check in with myself again, what do I think, feel and sense now? Also, what is happening between me and the supervisee? I feel that the ability to do this is important, not just in supervision, but in any situation involving clients. True empathy involves the ability to immerse ourselves in the experience of the other, but without losing ourselves in the process. Benner and Wrubel talk about how nurses need to enter patients' 'phenomenological field', which I take to mean stepping into their reality and seeing the world from their point of view, but again without forgetting who you are yourself (Benner & Wrubel 1989). I experience this constant shift in the focus of awareness as a very subtle 'in–out–in–out' movement, which is often paired with something physical such as a deeper in-breath, a slight hand movement or a brief look away.

HELICOPTER SKILLS

Hawkins and Shohet talk about the supervisor needing 'helicopter skills' (Hawkins & Shohet 2000:44). Think about that for a moment: what can a helicopter do? It can dart backwards and forwards, up and down; similarly, as supervisors we need to be able to shift our focus as required, but at the same time holding the overall situation in mind. So there is a continuous dialogue going on, between the supervisee and me and between me and my internal supervisor. All this may sound complicated and yet most of what I am talking about happens naturally; with experience we 'just do it', in the same way that after some lessons we 'just drive' without consciously needing to think 'right, first I'll look in the mirror, then I'll push in the clutch, then I'll … etc.'

The supervisee, on her part, often engages in an in–out movement too. As she talks about the client, she senses how that feels in the here and now, reflects on that, then takes it back to what that might say about the client, and so on. It is good for supervisors to encourage such 'self-supervision skills' as part of facilitating the development of the internal supervisor in supervisees. 'What are you feeling as you talk about this client?' I may ask, bringing the focus onto the here and now. Or, 'How does it feel to be in the room with this client?', shifting the focus to the 'there and then'.

As we reflect on the client, issue or situation in this way, clarity and meaning may gradually emerge.

SKILLS FOR FACILITATING REFLECTION

The value of musing and thinking about what is presented and how it is presented cannot be over-emphasised. Not only is this crucial in order to get a sense of the material that the supervisee brings, it is also useful for supervisees to see the reflective process in action. It is good for supervisees to see the supervisor thinking, checking hunches, testing hypotheses or checking the evidence (Bramley 1996:46). Not only is this good role-modelling, it also normalises the whole supervision process and does much to strengthen the relationship. It also contributes to cementing the working alliance. In effect, both supervisor and supervisee are thinking and working together on what is going on 'out there' as well as on what is happening 'in here' and what light this may throw on the 'supervision question'. The more relaxed you are and the less energy you spend on trying to be a good supervisor, the more you are likely to notice, which in turn will make you more effective.

However, facilitating someone to reflect is not always as easy as it sounds. It is good to help the supervisee reflect on questions such as:

- How did you feel at the time?
- How did you feel afterwards?
- How do you feel now that you are talking about it?
- How did you know how you felt?
- How would you like to have felt?
- How do you think your client felt?
- On what do you base this?
- How would you like your client to have felt?

And so on.

However, if we fire too many questions, the supervisee may feel that we are being too directive or that they are being interrogated, particularly if they are already feeling insecure and unsure of themselves. Reflecting, paraphrasing or summarising is helpful in encouraging the supervisee to say more (van Ooijen 2000:86–87). Other useful comments are: 'Tell me more', 'Go on, what else?', 'Can you explain that a bit further?' And so on. Sometimes encouraging comments like these are enough to help a supervisee to reflect deeper, particularly if they are experienced reflectors. Frequently, however, even very experienced people need additional help, as it tends to be precisely those issues they find difficult or are stuck with that are brought to supervision. Deeper reflection may be facilitated by saying something like:

- 'I sense there is something else going on'. Or
- 'I get the feeling that there is something blocking us here'. Or
- 'I could be wrong but I have the sense that we are missing something'. Or
- 'I don't think we have quite got to whatever is behind all this yet'.

And so on.

SUPPORTIVE CHALLENGE

The purpose of challenge, according to Page and Wosket is to 'open up areas for investigation' (Page & Wosket 2001:120). However, no matter how experienced we are, challenge and confrontation are never easy. How we challenge each other is therefore important, as an overly enthusiastic challenge could be experienced as an attack. This would defeat the purpose, as it is likely to have the effect of the supervisee becoming defensive, rather than opening herself up in order to look at her practice in a different way. Challenge often involves blind spots; by definition we are not aware of our blind spots and we may not like what we see once we become aware of them. Supportive challenge therefore first focuses on the person and ensures that they are valued for who they are as well as for their work, whilst encouraging them to reflect deeper or to reflect on a hitherto neglected area.

For example, a supervisor might say 'It seems that you were spot on when you said to the client...I wonder though what prevented you from taking this further?' Or, 'I have always noticed how good you are at keeping time boundaries. Here, though, you appear to find it difficult to end sessions on time. I am wondering what the reason for this might be?' Or, 'I do really value your honesty in the way you present your work, just now though I have the feeling that there is something that you are not saying ...'

Sometimes there are feelings just below the surface that the supervisee may be a bit hesitant to disclose, but that are potentially very useful to look at. Before diving in you need to be sure that the relationship you have with the supervisee is good and the reflective alliance sound, so that your supervisee feels safe enough to say things that may feel a bit delicate or difficult. Ways in which supervisees may be encouraged to do so may include asking questions regarding what fantasies come to mind when they think about the other person, how they feel when they are talking with them, or what hunches or hypotheses they have about the client.

CONCLUSION

The focus of this chapter is on what to do once the focus for the supervision has been determined. Helpful skills, qualities and tasks were discussed as well as the importance of creating plenty of space for reflection. Co-creation of meaning was held up as a desirable aim, rather than telling supervisees what to do. At the end of the chapter I introduced the idea that sometimes feelings may lie just below the surface, but can be brought to light provided the working alliance is good and the supervisor sensitive. 'What lies below the surface' is in fact the focus of the next chapter where I discuss ways of working with unconscious processes.

Questions for further reflection

- How do you currently help your supervisees to reflect?

- What, in your experience, is the difference between developmental and consultative supervision?

- What, if anything, would you like to change, in the way you give or receive supervision?

6

Working with the non-rational in the 'how' section

Fear is the first natural enemy a man must overcome on his path to knowledge. (Castaneda 1990:51)

Although most of us like to think of ourselves as rational human beings, in reality much of what we do is fuelled more by our feelings and emotions than we realise. In this chapter I first introduce the idea that much happens 'below the surface' of our everyday experience, before going on to discuss how we can work with the 'non-rational' parts of ourselves.

WORKING WITH THE NON-RATIONAL

Perhaps you thought while reading the previous chapter, what is the point of all this? Well, reflection does not just involve logic or common sense, it also involves the non-rational, those parts of ourselves that work differently. Much of what goes on in human interaction is not rational. So, therefore, when in supervision we try to make sense of such interactions we cannot solely depend on rational thought and methods, we need something else.

THE IDEA OF AN UNCONSCIOUS MIND

More happens in human interactions than can be accounted for by common sense. (Driver & Martin 2002)

In my experience people often switch off as soon as they hear the term 'psychodynamic', dismissing it as 'too complicated', or 'only

'Tip of the iceberg' view of consciousness

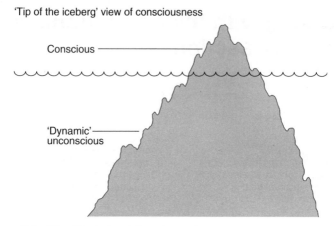

Figure 6.1 'Tip of the iceberg' view of consciousness.

concerned with what happened in the past'. As far as supervision is concerned, the basic assumption of the psychodynamic approach is the existence of a dynamic unconscious. I find it helpful to compare the mind to an iceberg: a small part is visible, but a much larger part remains hidden (see Fig. 6.1). When a boat meets an iceberg, the encounter does not only happen above the water (as the Titanic found to its cost). Similarly, whenever two or more people meet, the interaction that takes places happens at a conscious as well as an unconscious level (above and below the surface of the water). So whatever work we do, much happens between us and others that is not immediately apparent, but which can nevertheless have a huge effect.

HOW WE PROCESS EMOTION

Langs suggests that the human mind has evolved a dual system for the processing of emotion – one conscious, the other unconscious – which work in parallel (Langs 1994:21). By natural selection the conscious system evolved to deal with the issue of survival, both individually and as a species. It is therefore concerned with anything that threatens our life or safety as well as the more everyday search for food, shelter or friends. So the conscious system deals with the things that are obvious and can easily be perceived. This keeps it fully occupied, Langs suggests, and to add anything else would overload the system and therefore threaten our survival.

However, in any situation there is much more going on than simply getting food or building a shelter. The modern equivalent of that would be to go to the supermarket and to ensure that we have enough in our bank account to pay the rent or mortgage. We do not just go about our lives like machines or vulcans, devoid of any emotion. Every situation, whether we realise it or not, carries an emotional charge and it is here that the unconscious system becomes involved. It has the task of processing those emotions that would overload the coping mechanisms of the conscious system. The consequence of this is that we experience the world at two levels – one conscious and one unconscious. Often the experience of the two systems is very different and even in conflict with each other.

SCIENTIFIC EVIDENCE

Recent neurobiological research appears to back the importance of emotion and the concept of an unconscious mind. It seems that the two parts of our brain do not develop at the same rate, but that the right hemisphere develops first, very early on in life, after which it 'mediates the functional development of the unconscious mind' (Schore 2001).

Also, the neurologist Damassio discovered not only that emotion is necessary for rational thought, but also that body sensations cue the awareness of emotions. In other words, our emotions are based on body sensations and are themselves the basis for cognitive acts such as 'weighing consequences, deciding direction or identifying preferences' (Rothschild 2000:60).

Our perceptions are coloured by an inner world, of which we are largely unaware ... (Lomas 2001:1)

As we go about our daily lives, we are continually bombarded by one emotional stimulus after another. In order to protect the coping mechanisms of the conscious system from this even further (and perhaps to give the unconscious system time for processing), we evolved a raft of additional protective mechanisms, the so-called defence mechanisms. These include denial, avoidance, repression or distortions in the way we perceive things (Langs 1994:23). There are costs and benefits to this system. On the one hand, it helps us go about our everyday lives; on the other hand, it means that many of us are completely out of touch with what is going on inside us. The result of this is that consciously we are not very well adapted to learn from emotionally charged situations. The unconscious system's capacity for learning and adaptation, on the other hand, is virtually limitless. It has its own means of perceiving subliminal or unconscious messages, which are always to do with the here and now of any situation (Langs 1994:28). In other words, in any situation we unconsciously perceive messages lying beneath conscious interactions, which are often concerned with the context rather than the content. As Langs puts it, our 'unconscious system is continuously processing the conditions under which [a] discussion is taking place ...' (Langs 1994:29).

NOT SUCH A STRANGE IDEA?

The idea of unconscious processes and the thought that the world and our perception of it may not be as it seems can feel scary. I find that people sometimes react with angry resistance. To think that we know the world and then have someone telling us that it is different to what we thought may seem frightening, as if the rug of certainty is pulled from under us. And yet, is it really such a strange idea? If we ponder a bit on it we may realise that we are much more familiar with the idea of unconscious processes than we thought.

For example, the phenomenon of public relations did not start until the beginning of the last century, when Edward Bernaise (Freud's nephew) took the idea of his uncle – that there is a dynamic unconscious – seriously. He thought, 'If it does not just apply to people with neurosis but to everyone, how can I use it to sell products?' As a recent television programme (British Broadcasting Corporation 2002) showed, he is credited with single-handedly having sold the idea to women that smoking is a desirable thing to do. How? By getting women dressed up as suffragettes to appear at an important event smoking cigarettes. From then on smoking came unconsciously to be associated with being free and unconventional. Bernaise had banked on the idea that even the most conventional of us would harbour a secret wish to be the opposite. He was right. Women began to smoke in their millions and are still doing so today. It is perhaps a salutary thought that the idea that we have an unconscious mind is behind corporations spending millions on advertising and that it does work. Of course, consciously we know that buying a particular gravy cube does not make us a domestic goddess, or that a certain chewing gum will get not get us the girl. But that does not matter. As Langs states, the conscious and the unconscious mind are parallel systems and, even if consciously we think it is all a load of rubbish, it is likely that we are unconsciously affected all the same.

To take a more everyday example. We are all familiar with the idea of 'sleeping on it', when we have a problem, as often things seem better or clearer in the morning. Most of the time absolutely nothing has actually happened to change the situation, so why should we feel differently? In Langs's terms, although the situation itself has not changed, our view of it has. Somehow, while we were asleep, we continued to work on it, made sense of it and perhaps sorted things out.

Let me give an example from my own experience. Whenever I have an essay or article to write, workshop to plan or project to do, I think about it a bit, most of the time only having a very vague notion of what I might want to do, and then 'consciously' forget about it. Yet, when the time comes for me to sit down and actually do it, it often happens that a more or less fully formed idea appears in my mind. It is almost as if a seed that had been sown in my unconscious had slowly been incubating and developing, without me actually thinking about it at all, until it was ready to emerge.

It seems to me that the mind can function a bit like a computer in that it can be given one job to do while it continues to do another. As far as the idea of an unconscious mind is concerned, all we have to assume is that the brain can process emotional responses out of awareness, while we get on with our daily life. So it is really very efficient and perhaps not unlike the hard disc of a computer suddenly starting to update itself without being commanded to do so, while you are working on something else. The logical conclusion of all this is that we have emotional attitudes to things that we are not aware of, but which nevertheless influence our behaviour. However, with help it is possible to become aware of them. If we accept the premise that, in any interaction there is a great deal going on under the surface, then it follows that we would do ourselves and our work a disservice if we did not attempt to find out what that might be.

HOW CAN WE USE THE IDEA OF AN UNCONSCIOUS MIND IN SUPERVISION?

> *Nobody can know his or her own unconscious without help from some other person.* (Casement 1985:2)

In supervision we can gain clarity on what happens between ourselves and others, so that we do not get trapped in unhelpful patterns, either of our own or those of our clients, but can work creatively and effectively. Transference, counter-transfeence and parallel process are useful phenomena that can help us to do so.

TRANSFERENCE

Looking at transference and counter-transference phenomena is useful, both for illuminating the internal world of the client and for the further personal development of the supervisee. It is a 'natural human dynamic', as natural as 'breathing, eating and drinking' (Gilbert & Evans 2000:48).

Elements of transference enter in all relationships to a greater or lesser degree (Mandler 2000:23). Basically, it means that we tend to develop an idea or illusion about the people we meet, which is in some way a repetition of a relationship we had with someone in our past. This means that we do not necessarily see people objectively, but experience them through our own subjective filter, which is constructed out of our past experiences. In other words, we 'project' elements that belong to someone in the past onto someone we are in relationship with now (van Ooijen 2000:165). In a way this is not surprising; how else would we make sense of the world? However, if we stay in the grip of transference, this will get in the way of our seeing people for who they actually are. We have put them in a box as it were, and become closed to any other possibilities. None of this happens consciously; therefore, in our work with clients it is useful to help them to unravel their transference reactions to us as well as to others.

COUNTER-TRANSFERENCE

> *Transference phenomena may be seen as manifestations of an unmet developmental need and may therefore provide useful clues for understanding the client's inner world.*
> (Gilbert & Evans 2000:7)

There are not many people who have not had some kind of deficit in their development. Therefore, no matter how mature or experienced we are as practitioners, we remain vulnerable. When something triggers off that 'gap' in our development, our 'script button' gets pressed, and we may 'react' as that child we once were, rather than as the mature professional we are today. When we find ourselves acting out of character it is therefore useful to look at the client's projections in order to find out whether they somehow hook into our own history.

So clients do not have the monopoly on transference reactions, professionals develop them too. In supervision we can be helped to tease out not only our clients' transference reactions but those that belong to us as well, in which case we speak of 'counter-transference'. Strictly speaking, the term implies a process by which we unconsciously 'counter' anything that has been 'transferred' onto us by another (van Ooijen 2000:168). However, as the discussion above indicates, it is all a bit more complicated than that. For simplicity's sake, however, whatever the client experiences is called transference, whereas anything experienced by the practitioner is called counter-transference. Counter-transference has been called 'an instrument of research into the patient's unconscious' (Heimann 1950:75). By this Heimann means that we can learn to be alert to our own experiences as they can give useful clues to what might be going on for the other person.

 EXAMPLE

A supervisee reported that she had a client she kept 'forgetting'. She would look in her diary, see the person's initials and then not remember who it was she was supposed to see in that particular time slot. One day we had agreed that she would present an overview of her current workload. She looked at her list of clients, and on seeing the name of this particular client could not remember who she was. When we reflected on this it seemed that there was something about this client that she had not yet seen, but that needed to be brought to light. The supervisee's constant 'forgetting' the client thus served as a useful pointer to the work that needed to happen.

Of course transference and counter-transference reactions can also happen between supervisor and supervisee and can be very useful to bring to awareness (Hawkins & Shohet 2000:64).

Using a 'transference filter'

Unless your workload is very small, you cannot bring every client to supervision every time. It is therefore useful to develop an 'internal supervisor'. By this I mean a sense within ourselves, something that observes what is going on between me and the client, as if I was discussing it in a supervision session. The development of this sense is not easy; it needs constant attention and will probably never be completed. For example, I often find that, as soon as the client has left, I realise the significance of something he said. I also find it interesting to read my process notes through a transference filter. By this I mean that, just for practice, I read everything that happened between me and the client as an expression of transference. I am often surprised just how significant seemingly ordinary statements can seem when looked at in this way. I am not saying that everything in a session is an expression of transference, although people with a pure psychodynamic orientation may well hold this view. What I am saying is that it is an interesting way in which to develop that observing sense that constitutes an 'internal supervisor' (Gilbert & Evans 2000:48).

 EXAMPLE

A client was talking about his dental treatment. This was ongoing and expensive, but although the painful infections he had been suffering were now less frequent, the problem had not yet disappeared completely. When, in the next session, I checked out whether he perhaps felt like this about the counselling too, this was indeed the case. In fact, he had been thinking of leaving, but my recognition of how he was feeling reassured him and he decided to continue seeing me.

PARALLEL PROCESS

Supervisor: You know, I was struck by your posture and tone of voice as you talked.

Supervisee: (surprised) What do you mean?

Supervisor: Well, you slumped like this (demonstrated) and your voice was very monotonous. (Supervisor spoke the last words in a monotonous voice.)

Supervisee: Really? I had no idea, gosh, that is interesting.

Supervisor: Does your client speak like that?

And so on.

Parallel process is an extremely interesting phenomenon where the supervisee somehow behaves like her client, without being aware that she is doing so. Although it may seem a bizarre idea, parallel process is in fact very common, and probably happens because something about the client has not yet been processed. In a way it is as if we have eaten something rather heavy which is still lying on our stomach, undigested. In other words, the unprocessed bit of the client is brought into the supervision room (vomited up), in the hope that the supervision will help the 'digestion'. Parallel process is a way whereby the supervisee unconsciously brings the client into the here and now of the supervision situation. This is very helpful as it gives the supervisor a chance to really get a sense of the person being talked about. Clues to parallel process are supervisee behaviours that are somehow surprising, out of character or in some other way different than usual.

 EXAMPLE

A supervisee related how a person she was working with never showed any emotion. The client was always very rational and tended to make light of things. On this particular occasion the supervisee related a story told by the client. As she did so I started to feel immensely sad. When I checked this out with the supervisee she said that she too felt sad, but had never felt this before when she was with this client. It was as if she had taken the material into the supervision session, all nicely wrapped up, thus paralleling how the client brought his material to her. In giving it attention in the supervision, however, the parcel was beginning to become undone, and the sadness was spilling out. Having this information was very useful for the supervisee, as it helped her to understand the magnitude of the feeling. She felt that the reason why the client was so diligent in keeping the parcel wrapped up was for fear of being overwhelmed.

The phenomenon of parallel process is very useful because it brings the client into the room, which helps the supervisor to get a sense of the client. The phenomenon can also be helpful when a practitioner feels stuck, as sometimes she is caught in the same stuckness as the client. If the supervisor then reflects this back to the supervisee it can help her realise that the stuckness belongs to the client, not to her, which can sometimes be sufficient to overcome it.

METHODS FOR WORKING WITH THE NON-RATIONAL

Working with the non-rational in supervision is very helpful for counsellors and other mental health professionals. However, I find that the various techniques can also be illuminating in other types of supervision, situations and relationships.

I like the idea of keeping things light, of working with the non-rational in a playful way. Supervision has been referred to as a 'play space' (Hawkins & Shohet 2000:7). Also, Bollas suggests that ideas can be pushed backwards and forwards and talks about 'releasing the subjective mind into play' (Bollas 1987:206).

The basic idea in psychodynamic work is that healing occurs not so much through aiming to fix, cure, or change, but in being deeply understood. The helping process therefore involves facilitating clients to really get to know themselves, in the hope that this will help them to make changes when they are ready.

The task of the supervisor therefore involves facilitating the practitioner's understanding in two main areas:

- What is going on for the client?
- What is happening in the relationship between practitioner and client and how helpful is this?

As discussed earlier in the chapter these questions can be addressed by focusing on the there and then (the Therapy Matrix) or by focusing on the here and now (the Supervision Matrix), but good supervision probably involves both areas (Hawkins & Shohet 2000).

HELPFUL STRATEGIES

Hawkins and Shohet suggest a number of helpful strategies to bring to light transference and counter-transference dynamics between the supervisee and their client. For example:

- Imagine yourself on a desert island with your client … what happens?
- Who does this client remind you of?
- If you were a fly sitting on the wall, what would you see? (Hawkins & Shohet 2000:75–80)

I encourage you, the reader, to come up with similar ideas yourself, as it is good to have quite a repertoire. Here are some more ideas:

- If you were both cars, what kind of car would you be?

You could then go on to ask questions such as:

- What happens when you are both waiting for the traffic lights to go green? Or,
- You are both in a race, what happens?

You can play about with this kind of question and substitute cars by animals, fish, plants, insects, furniture, boats, whatever you can think of really. Or you may like to ask, 'If your work with this client was part of a novel, how would it continue?' You can then brainstorm different versions of the plot.

Other methods include asking:

- What does it feel like to be in the room with this client? Or,
- Think of your client for a few moments, focus on how your body feels – what might this be telling you, can you give it a name, a colour, an image?
- If your client was an animal, a fish, a plant, a car, a colour – what would it be? Can you say a bit more about the reason for your choice?
- Imagine a treasure hunt – what would be the client's treasure?

It is also useful to ask the supervisee what the client could be searching for (unconsciously). Or who they imagine the client needs them to be.

As far as transference and counter-transference between supervisor and supervisee is concerned, it is good for both to be up-front regarding any images, fantasies, feelings or bodily sensations that occur. It is only when these are 'put on the table' that they are available for reflection. Not all experiences we have when in the room with a supervisee are to do with them or the material they bring; some of it may be entirely generated by ourselves. However, time and again I find that, even if something does not seem significant, putting it out there for us to look at is very helpful.

Creative methods

Playful methods such as those suggested above can really free up things. Creative ways of working such as those suggested in Chapter 4 for use in Step 1 could also be helpful in Step 2 as they can help a supervisee reflect more deeply on something. This is because they can help us access these areas of the brain that deal with emotion and feeling. Sometimes we use words to hide behind rather than to clarify, but playful creative ways of working can offer a more direct route to what may be below the surface. People often find that as they write, paint or draw they actually reflect as they go along. Somehow using a medium other than talking seems to help people to highlight different aspects of a situation.

Taking the role of the client

The supervisee can be interviewed as if he is his client and asked questions such as:

- What is going on for her?
- What are her hopes for the work with the supervisee?
- What might she be hoping for unconsciously?
- How might she be subverting the work with the supervisee?
- How does she feel about the relationship with the supervisee?
- What would she like the supervisee to do/be?
- How would that be?

Alternatively, the supervisee could be asked to 'rapid write' the answers. (Rapid writing involves writing whatever comes to mind without first thinking about it and without stopping.) It can also be interesting to try writing the answers to the questions with the non-dominant hand; the answers can sometimes be quite different.

Another method involves asking the supervisee to 'be his client' and then convey in a word or image how he feels.

THINGS THAT CAN GO WRONG IN SUPERVISION

When something goes wrong in supervision it is crucial to re-examine the relationship in order to find out what is happening.

 EXAMPLE

A supervisor had noticed that his supervisee often tended to react to a searching question in a particular way, so one day he said, 'What I notice about you is that you tend to …' The supervisee became defensive and the session appeared at an impasse. The supervisor realised that this 'rupture' in the working alliance might have something to do with the way he had phrased things. When he asked the supervisee about this the supervisee said yes, she had felt that the comment was so generalised that it had made her feel judged. She felt that the supervisor was behaving like a detached observer, only interested in finding fault. They then talked about how they might do things differently. Their discussion helped to repair the rupture. The supervisor was non-defensive, which helped the supervisee to let go of defences too.

In the above example it was the general nature of the comment that upset the supervisee rather than what was pointed out. If the supervisor had said 'What happened just now?', the question would have been in context and the supervisee would have had a chance to respond.

As supervision is about a relationship, it is useful to ask ourselves what we have contributed if things have gone wrong. For example, if a supervisee seems rebellious or uninterested or unreliable regarding actually turning up, it is time to examine ourselves. Thus the controlling supervisor may constellate the rebellious supervisee, the all-knowing supervisor the insecure supervisee, the overly helpful supervisor the dependent supervisee, and so on. Therefore, when things have gone wrong and we discern a certain unhelpful behaviour in our supervisee, it is time to ask ourselves, 'What is its opposite and has this somehow found a home in me, and if so how has this happened?'

GAMES PEOPLE PLAY IN SUPERVISION

Things often go wrong because either one or both parties are playing one of the following games.

Who is the best practitioner?   Whatever the supervisee says, the supervisor will find a better way of dealing with it. In effect the supervisor is being competitive with the supervisee, which can lead to telling the supervisee what to do, rather than helping them develop their own way. The opposite is also possible in that the supervisee may refuse to take on board anything the supervisor says, feeling that they know better.

My model is better than yours   This can happen with practitioners who do not share the same theoretical orientation. For example, the supervisor may attempt to impose their model of working rather than validating the supervisee's own model and help her work within that. Alternatively, the supervisee may dismiss whatever the supervisor says as 'not relevant'.

Become my ideal   The supervisor wants the supervisee to confirm to her vision of an 'ideal' counsellor, nurse, occupational therapist or whatever. This is often based on how the supervisor thinks she is herself or would like to be.

What mistakes have you made this week?   Particularly where the supervision has a managerial element there can be a tendency to focus too much on looking for mistakes. This may well be for positive reasons, such as a sense of responsibility for the well-being of the client or the quality of the service. Whereas it is obviously important to ascertain that people work within their professional ethical codes, over-emphasis on what has been done wrong and a corresponding failure to value good work can make people feel undermined as professionals. Ultimately it is demotivating and can have the opposite effect to what it is designed to achieve – to maintain and enhance good practice.

I won't mention it if you won't – collusion   Here the supervisor does not confront a supervisee with poor practice, what Page and Wosket call the 'passively optimistic' style of supervision (Page & Wosket 2001:25).

I'll try and work with your client through you   Rather than helping the supervisee to reflect and thus further develop their work with someone, the supervisor attempts to work with the client vicariously. This means that they only focus on what might be going on for the client and what has been done, after which they will suggest what they think should happen. In effect, the supervisee does not get a look in and the importance of the relationship between the supervisee and their client is ignored. The supervisee may end up feeling deskilled or undermined, very frustrated and angry, or a combination of all of these.

I will have the answers for whatever you don't know   Here the supervisor feels that they have to know all the answers, which is bound to create either dependency or frustration in their supervisees.

Become like me and you will be all right   Here a supervisor bolsters her self-esteem by wanting her supervisees to be just like her. This will hold up not only her supervisees' development but her own as well (Corbett in Kugler 1995:65).

I need your adoration to make me feel better   The less experienced the supervisee the more unequal the relationship is likely to be, and the greater the temptation on the supervisor to abuse their power. Gilbert & Evans (2000:109) call this 'disciple hunting' and say that it can be extremely subtle and is not always easy to spot. What it comes down to, however, is that the supervisee is made to feel that they cannot manage on their own as all their ideas are ultimately derived from the supervisor.

THE METAPHOR OF THE SHADOW

The 'shadow' is a Jungian metaphor for our own dark side. When the sun shines, it does not just create a pool of light, it also creates a shadow. Also, as it happens, the more intense the light (as in the summer), the darker the shadow will be. We all have a dark and a light side to our personalities. It is not easy for us to tolerate the tension between dark and light, which often leads us to repress our negative side. However, it will continue to exist and operate from within our unconscious. So the more we ignore it, the more likely it becomes that eventually it will surface in a destructive manner. (Perhaps it is this that has led some practitioners to actually kill patients.)

THINKING POINT

Think of someone who does not like you. What do they say about you? What are your feelings regarding them? What might it mean? Now try to imagine that you are asked to give an opinion on someone else, what kind of person are they? What do you think about them as a professional? It may be useful to discuss your thoughts with someone you trust.

The shadow in supervision

Taking on the role of supervisor brings with it many temptations, some of which are outlined in the above 'games'. It has been suggested that the motivation to work in a helping profession is often highly ambiguous (Guggenbuhl-Craig 1996:10). Ironically, the more altruistic and dedicated we are, the more likely we are to fall into our 'power shadow' (Guggenbuhl-Craig 1996:17). I certainly admit that I have fallen into this shadow myself on several occasions and no doubt will be tempted to do so again. It can be very hard when you think that you know better than anyone else does what should happen – for the good of the clients, naturally – not to impose that view. And yet, that is pure grandiosity. None of us have all the answers, and in supervision our task is to help the supervisee achieve the clarity that will enable them to provide the best possible service for their clients. Whatever that may turn out to be might be quite different than if we were working with the same people, but nevertheless just as (or even more) effective.

The power shadow may look different according to the practitioner's profession. It may be helpful to look at the stereotypes that exist (positive as well as negative) for that profession as clues to the power shadow may often be found there (Guggenbuhl-Craig 1996:30).

The following example was related to me by a workshop participant.

EXAMPLE: THE 'GURU'

One counselling supervisor always suggested ways of saying a particular thing to clients. Whereas these suggestions were usually helpful, the supervisee felt increasingly irritated by them. 'It just does not allow me to develop my own way of doing things,' she said. Suggesting how to do or say things can sometimes be helpful, particularly with supervisees who are still fairly inexperienced in their profession. However, the aim of supervision should be to help the supervisee to develop her own way of working. In the above example it appeared that the supervisor's failure to do so was inhibiting the supervisee's professional growth. What happened in this case was that the supervisee frequently found herself unable to recall any of the supervisor's suggestions, despite always dutifully writing them down. 'Why do you think that is?' I asked. 'Because I am treated as a passive, empty vessel,' she answered. 'I need to be actively involved in things in order to remember them; being given such concrete suggestions reminds me too much of school and homework. It brings out the rebellious side in me.'

This was a salutary conversation for me, as I knew that I too have on occasion erred on the side of giving too much. Partly this is because of enthusiasm and of wanting the best for supervisees and their clients. But, if I am honest, there is probably also a hint of the power shadow in action, wanting to impress, to shine, to be looked up to – and it is this that in the long run is so off-putting as it serves the needs of the supervisor rather than those of the supervisee.

When we have fallen into our power shadow we need to 'look it in the eye' (Guggenbuhl-Craig 1996:30). If I, as a supervisor, have fallen into my shadow, I need to admit this once I realise what has happened, no matter how painful this may be. Not only will this help repair the working alliance, it is also good role-modelling as it will help the supervisee to do the same if they, for their part, fall into their power shadow with their clients.

We may not like to admit to things having gone wrong for fear of loss of face or credibility, but the opposite is actually the case.

By showing the supervisee that we are not afraid to admit to mistakes and lapses of awareness, we help the supervisee to do the same. It also helps to reduce the power differential and lessen the likelihood of it happening again. The supervisee can be enlisted to watch out with us for similar lapses in the future and point them out when they occur. Sometimes a supervisee may be uncomfortable with this, as they want to see the supervisor as all-knowing and without fault. Whereas such a supervisee can be flattering to the ego, they are bad for the soul. In such a case it is necessary to investigate with the supervisee what this may be about. It would seem important for training programmes to include facilitating practitioners to become aware of their own dark sides and the 'many ways in which the shadow sides of their chosen work can express themselves' (Guggenbuhl-Craig 1996:153). It may be good, from time to time, to ask ourselves the question 'What is it that made me choose this profession?' Or, 'Why do I want to be a supervisor?' Or even, 'Why have I decided to write about supervision?' It is likely that the answer is a mixture of positive and negative reasons, of dark and of light – and this is reality, this is what life is like. What is important is that we do not remain ignorant of this but are willing to question our own motives, rather than denying them. So, it is not about eliminating the negative, as this will only help it go underground, but about awareness. If we are helped to become aware of our own shadow we are much less likely to act upon it. Ironically, it is very difficult to see our own shadow, our own blind spots. Our own supervision can be helpful here as well as our enemies! It can be useful to find out why some people do not like us – they may see the very thing that we are blind to in ourselves! (Guggenbuhl-Craig 1996:28–29). Also, the methods outlined in the section 'working with the non-rational' are excellent in teasing out the shadow wherever it occurs.

CONCLUSION

In this chapter I discussed the 'how' rather than the 'what' of an intervention, the supervisee's feelings about the situation, client or intervention and the supervisee's impressions of the thoughts and feelings of the client or relevant others. The supervisory relationship itself is a useful vehicle through which practitioners' work with clients may be examined. Much of what happens between people occurs at an unconscious level, which is why it is useful to pay attention to 'non-rational' ways of working. These methods are also helpful in facilitating our becoming aware of our own shadow. Lastly, the working alliance between supervisor and supervisee is crucial to the effectiveness of supervision. Both parties therefore need to be alert to the many ways in which things can go wrong and be prepared to 'put this on the table' so that difficulties can be discussed and overcome.

The next chapter will deal with what to do once it feels that the reflection has been completed.

Questions for further reflection

- Do you currently work with unconscious processes?

- If so, what methods do you use?

- If not, would you now consider some of the methods discussed in this chapter?

7

Moving forward in supervision: working with the 'what now' of supervision

... learning was the most difficult task a man could undertake ... I had wanted to find it without doing any work because I had expected him to hand out all the information. If he had done so, he said, I would never have learned. (Castaneda 1990:54)

... it is not sufficient to just 'do'. I must also reflect on my own process of doing ... (Holloway 1995:xiii)

 EXAMPLE: THE OUTCOME OF SUPERVISION CAN BE SURPRISING

'It sounds as if you are working really well with this client,' a supervisor said to his supervisee. The supervisee was surprised to hear this: 'Sometimes you get so used to the way you are working that you forget what it is that you are doing,' she said. They had just reflected on her work with a client and the supervision had helped her to make conscious what she was doing automatically. Whereas there is nothing wrong with unconscious competence, it can be really helpful to make it conscious from time to time. The supervisee had felt that she was at a loss with this client and that she did not really know what she was doing. Having reflected on her work it appeared that what she was doing was fine. She now realised that her feelings were probably a reflection of how her client was feeling. This realisation then helped her to see a way forward with this client.

In Step 3 the supervisor first helps the supervisee to clarify and consolidate what has been achieved in Step 2. This can be described as a 'reflection on the reflection'. The supervisee is then helped to move from reflection to action, which involves clarifying how the new insights can be used in future work. This will include ensuring that these actions are ethical and constitute 'best practice'. The effectiveness of both the process and the content of supervision is evaluated and a record is kept of the session as part of the 'evidence' of the effectiveness of the supervision.

In this chapter, I first consider the five tasks involved in Step 3: learning, action, monitoring, evaluating and evidence. Next I focus on the evaluation of the effectiveness of supervision over time, as well as how to use the 3-Step method to keep a record of supervision sessions. In the last part of the chapter, I discuss how to end a supervisory relationship.

THE FIVE TASKS OF STEP 3 – LAMEE

In Step 3 the focus is on five factors: learning, action, monitoring, evaluation and providing evidence. I like to use the acronym LAMEE to remind me of these. In Table 7.1 I set out some useful supervisory tasks under each of the five headings.

I will go through each of the five tasks in turn and discuss how the supervisor and the supervisee can work together to achieve these important tasks. Although the tasks as set out in Table 7.1 may seem daunting, in practice many supervisory couples are probably already doing most if not all of them. However if, like me, you have a tendency to get really interested in what is being discussed, it is quite possible to get so taken up with the excitement of whatever issue you are reflecting on that it is easy to forget what needs to be achieved. Sometimes people find that they have nearly reached the end of the session and they are only halfway through their reflection. Now it is true that sometimes this cannot be helped, as some issues need more than one session. However, for much of the time it is quite possible to achieve clarity quite quickly, provided a structure is adhered to and you know what it is that you want to achieve. I believe that Step 3 is an important part of supervision and deserves to be given due attention. The LAMEE acronym may provide a useful aide memoire – indeed a structure for this part of the supervision session.

Table 7.1 Step 3: tasks of the 'what now' section

	Supervisor	Supervisee
Learning	Help the supervisee to be clear on her thoughts, feelings and views Help the supervisee to describe her new 'super' vision Help the supervisee to be clear on what has been learnt Help the supervisee to know what is still not clear and may need more thought	Clarifying and consolidation of the reflection in Step 2 Develop greater insight and awareness
Action	Help the supervisee to find ways of linking the reflection to action Facilitate the supervisee to brainstorm regarding possible actions if appropriate	Linking the reflection to action Generating ideas for action Planning action Decision-making
Monitoring	Facilitate effective and ethical practice Promote 'best' practice and confront bad practice	Act upon the 'super' vision
Evaluating	Evaluate the effectiveness of the session Check whether the goals identified in Step 1 have been achieved Reflect on the content of the supervision session Agree main themes and outcomes Reflect on the process of the supervision session Give and receive feedback on the process	Evaluate the effectiveness of the session Evaluate own process honestly Give and receive constructive feedback
Evidence	Keep notes of sessions as agreed with the supervisee	Keep notes of the session

LEARNING

- Help the supervisee to be clear on her thoughts, feelings and views.
- Help the supervisee to describe her new 'super' vision.
- Help the supervisee to be clear on what has been learnt.
- Help the supervisee to know what is still not clear and may need more thought.

The first task of Step 3 is to clarify and consolidate the reflection that took place at Step 2 in order to find out, not only what the supervisee thinks and feels now, but also what she has learnt. In other words, the task is to find out whether a 'super' vision has been achieved. This can be facilitated by asking questions such as:

- What do you think now?
- What do you feel now?
- How do you see things now?
- How is the way you see things now different from when we first started talking?
- What have you learnt?

Open-ended questions like this give the supervisee a chance to pull her thoughts together and articulate her new vision of things. Sometimes this means that there is a need to go back to Step 2 for a bit in order to reflect on an aspect that has been neglected or overlooked. Or, if there is no time, an agreement can be made to look at it next time if that seems appropriate and useful.

ACTION

- Help the supervisee to find ways of linking the reflection to action.
- Facilitate the supervisee to brainstorm regarding possible actions if appropriate.

Having identified what has been learnt, we next need to focus on what the supervisee wants to do with her new insight. It is not always necessary to plan specific action – sometimes a clearer view of a situation is in itself sufficient for change to occur. Indeed, change is not even always necessary, as was the case in the example given at the beginning of this chapter. Even if no specific action is required though, the clearer vision of the supervisee is bound to influence her actions.

In order to help the supervisee decide how best to use her new insight it is useful to ask questions such as:

- What is your plan for using the new insights you have gained?
- What action if any do you want to take now?
- What would you now like to do?
- What do you now 'not' want to do?

You will notice that all the questions are open-ended. Sometimes supervisors find it difficult to curb their impatience or enthusiasm at this stage and are tempted to say things like 'Why don't you do …' or 'What I would do if I were you is …'. However, this is not a good idea at all as it robs the supervisee of the chance to decide for himself what he needs to do. A very good skill or quality for supervisors to develop at Step 3 is the ability to be patient. However, if the supervisee is clear that he wants to do something but is having difficulty in deciding what action he wants to take, it can be helpful to ask questions such as:

- What do you think a person you admire might do?
- What have you done in similar situations in the past?
- What might you have wanted to do instead?
- What useful information have you gained from mistakes made in the past?

Helping the supervisee to come up with ideas

It can also be helpful to have a brainstorming session, with the supervisee generating as many ideas as possible. I like to do this by means of a 'spidergram'. I write the word 'action' in the centre of a large sheet of paper and draw a circle around it. Then I draw lines from this circle going in all directions, like the legs of a spider. The ideas developed during the brainstorm are written alongside the spider's legs (see Fig. 7.1).

When we seem to have come to a full stop I draw four more legs and invite the supervisee to think of two things they absolutely should not do and two ideas that are completely wacky. For example I may ask:

- What is the worst thing you could do?
- What is the one thing you must definitely not do?
- What is the craziest idea you can think of?

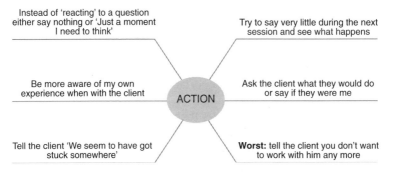

Figure 7.1 Example of a spidergram being used in a brainstorming session.

This process gives the supervisee a large number of ideas to work with. It seems that the 'must never do' and 'wacky' ideas somehow free up people's thinking, so that they come up with a solution quite quickly. Also, if it does not work then there are plenty of other ideas to think about. Once a good number of ideas have been generated, the supervisee needs to be helped to choose the action or actions most likely to have the desired outcome. In order to help the supervisee to do so it can help to ask questions such as:

- What is your preferred action(s)?
- Which action(s) do you think is most likely to be effective?

When the supervisee comes up with his preferred action or the one that is most likely to be effective (these may not necessarily be the same), it is useful to ask: 'What are your reasons for your choice?' This is in order to find out whether the supervisee has really learnt from the reflection and gained in understanding. If their rationale for the chosen action is well thought out and obviously based on the new insights gained at Step 2, and, above all, most likely to be of benefit to the client, then it is likely to be a good decision. It is not always easy to know what is the best action; I therefore discuss this issue further in the next chapter, where I apply the 3-Step method to ethical decision-making.

Sharing ideas, hunches and experience

Although I stressed the importance of allowing supervisees to develop their own insights and plans for action, it would be ungenerous if a supervisor did not share his ideas, hunches or experience, if this is appropriate. Although it is ideally the supervisee who develops ideas, actions and strategies, they frequently also like some help or alternative ideas that they have not thought of. In that case a supervisor could offer his suggestions, but in such a way that they are not seen as 'commands'. Offering more than one option and making it clear that these are only suggestions will prevent this from happening. If a supervisor is much more experienced than the supervisee, it is all the more important to facilitate the supervisee to come up with his own ideas first. At the same time, however, the function of supervision includes that of education (the educative or formative function). The skill at this stage is to facilitate the supervisee in an optimum way – helping them to come up with their own ideas, whilst at the same time teaching them what they need to know, but do not know already. In other words, the real skill here is to know when to sit back and when to come forward.

Checking out possible consequences of an action

Before an action is decided upon, its possible consequences need to be looked at. Even experienced practitioners may sometimes need to be reminded of this. In the next chapter I discuss the issue of consequences more fully, with particular reference to ethical decision-making. Below are a number of methods that may help in the teasing out of the possible consequences of an action.

Asking helpful questions

The most straightforward method is to ask the supervisee pertinent questions about the possible effects of what they are planning to do. Helpful questions to ask may include:

• What do you think the effect of that might be?
• How do you think your client will feel or react?
• What might the consequences be?
• How do you think that will be for you?
• If you were the client, how might you feel?

Trying the action out in role-play

It is always a good idea to try out possible actions in the supervision session itself. The supervisor can role-play the client and give feedback regarding the impact of the supervisee's action. Alternatively, the supervisee can role-play the client, with the supervisor taking the role of the supervisee. It can be useful to set a clear time limit for this in order not to get carried away and forget about the purpose of the role-play.

An advantage of trying things out like this is that any difficulties can be ironed out beforehand. Getting a sense of what it is like to be at the receiving end of an intervention is very helpful, as the effect is not always what is intended.

Visualising the action

Visualisation is another way of helping the supervisee to take the part of the client (or whichever person he has talked about in the session). The procedure is as follows:

1. Ask the supervisee to close his eyes.
2. Then ask him to imagine that he is the client, and is in the room with the supervisee.
3. Talk him through the planned action.
4. Ask him to sit with this for a minute or so to get a sense of how it feels.
5. Ask the supervisee to open his eyes and report back on his experience.

Rapid writing

Again, ask the supervisee to imagine himself in the place of his client and then to write down whatever it is that comes to mind without stopping to think about it. In other words, write rapidly and without interruption for 3 minutes. After the 3 minutes the written material can be used as a basis for further reflection on the possible consequences.

MONITORING

The role of monitoring is to:

- Facilitate effective and ethical practice.
- Promote 'best' practice and confront bad practice.

Monitoring supervisees' work is of course an ongoing task and is one of the three functions of supervision. However, it does not just apply to what they report they have done; it is also relevant to what they are planning to do – or even to what they are not doing but perhaps should do.

New supervisors can find the monitoring function of supervision the most difficult one as it may involve challenging the supervisee on something they have done, are planning to do, or are failing to carry out. However, it is an important function and if as a supervisor you are not happy with a supervisee's ongoing or planned actions, you, as her supervisor, do have a duty to take action. In the first instance this should involve working out the consequences of her actions as discussed above. Sometimes situations are very complicated and may need more unpacking. Particularly where the supervisee's work involves more than one person there may be conflict in that what is good for one person appears to be against the well-being of another person. If this is the case, the adapted 3-Step method discussed in Chapter 8 offers a way of working out what needs to be done.

If, having done this, you remain concerned about the supervisee's planned way of working, you need to discuss this with her openly and explain the reasons for your concern. Hopefully the supervisee will then agree, which will pave the way for working out what needs to be done between you. If, however, you and the supervisee disagree and you are convinced that her work is not in accordance with 'best practice' and ethical guidelines, then you need to inform her of what you are going to do about it. Fortunately it does not happen very often that a supervisor needs to take action herself because the supervisee cannot see what the problem is. Most of the time, supervisees are, in the final analysis, grateful that they have been helped to work ethically, and prefer to take whatever action is needed themselves. I always feel that this indicates great strength of character and needs to be supported. Very occasionally, though, it is necessary for a supervisor to take action because the supervisee refuses to do so. This is always extremely difficult and painful for all concerned. This type of situation also shows why we all need supervision, even those of us who supervise. So, if you are in this situation, do discuss it in your own supervision and get all the support you need.

Mistakes are valuable

As far supervisees are concerned, it can be difficult to realise that you have made a mistake or that it might have been better if you had done things differently. Finding this difficult is not wrong, it is part of being human. We all make mistakes – none of us is perfect. And, as I have stated elsewhere, mistakes are the ideal way in which we learn!

EVALUATING
Evaluate the effectiveness of the session

It seems crucial to me not to forget to check out how effective the supervision session has been for the supervisee. As a supervisor it is easy to think it has gone really well, only to discover later that the supervisee's experience was rather different. As the purpose of supervision is first and foremost to help supervisees achieve best practice, their experience of how well they feel facilitated in this is clearly all-important. No matter how good we feel our supervision is, if the supervisee does not experience it as such it is not as effective as it might be. Useful questions to check out the supervisee's experience regarding the session's effectiveness may include:

- How effective do you feel the session has been for you?
- What might have helped to make it more effective?
- What might we still need to look at?
- What have we not reflected on?
- What is still not clear?

Check whether the goals identified in Step 1 have been achieved

The perceived effectiveness of the session will be intricately bound up with whether or not the desired outcomes identified in Step 1 have been achieved. Sometimes supervisors (and perhaps the supervisees) get so interested in what they are talking about that they lose sight of the purpose of the session, or even of the supervision. Indeed, this can be a ploy by the supervisee to avoid having her practice looked at too closely. Some supervisees know exactly how to catch the interest of the supervisor and get him to talk about something he finds hard to resist. This kind of thing is bound to happen once in a while and is not necessarily wrong if the supervisee does find it genuinely helpful. However, if instead of reflecting on the supervisee's practice you find that you and your supervisee habitually talk about other issues, it may be time to take stock in order to find out not only what is happening, but also why it is happening and what is possibly being avoided.

The most straightforward way to check that the session has achieved what you set out to do is to ask the supervisee straight out: 'What about the outcomes of the session? We agreed that you wanted to … (here state the outcomes specifically). Tell me to what extent you feel that they have been achieved.'

I try to steer away from asking too many closed question such as 'Have we achieved the outcomes?' as that may make it more difficult for the supervisee to say 'No', or 'Not quite', or 'I am not sure.'

If the outcomes have not quite been achieved it will be necessary to check out why this is so. Indeed, the supervisee may be asked: 'What, do you think, are the reasons for us not achieving the goals?' If the supervisee feels that the outcomes were not achieved because of the way in which the session was conducted, you may like to go straight on to reflecting on the content as well as the process of the session as discussed below. Of course, it may also be the case that the goals were unrealistic, or that the issue is very complicated and therefore unlikely to be clarified in one session. In that case you may agree that both of you need to think about it some more and perhaps come back to it in a later session.

Reflect on the content of the supervision session – agree main themes and outcomes

In addition to ascertaining whether or not the goals identified in Step 1 have been achieved, it is also good to check what the actual content of the session consisted of and what other outcomes there might be. You may like to introduce this by making comments such as: 'So, what have we been talking about?' You can then both state what you feel the main themes were and perhaps make a note of this, either now or later.

Another useful question is: 'What, for you, are the outcomes of this session?' Again, these can be noted (as seen below) as they are part of the evidence of the session's effectiveness. You could also say: 'With hindsight, what other outcomes might you have wanted, that you did not think of before?'

This kind of question can help the supervisee become much clearer on what they themselves can do to get the most out of sessions. They may realise that adequate preparation for sessions is one of the best ways in which they can help make the supervision really work for them.

Reflect on the process of the supervision session – give and receive feedback on the process

Last but by no means least, it is important to check out with each other how you have felt during the session and to give each other feedback. Again, this can on occasion feel sticky; sometimes it may seem easier not to say anything and to hope that next time things will be better. I believe this is a mistake. Unless both supervisor and supervisee are honest with each other it is not possible to know how well you are working together. Moreover, unless you say what you are unhappy about, the other person is not going to know. Sometimes I hear people talking about their supervisors, how unhappy they are with them, and how they would like things to be different. I usually then say, 'Have you talked with them about it?' Quite often the answer is 'No I haven't actually – do you think I should?' The answer is 'Yes, most definitely'. Unless the supervision is felt to be helpful there is no point in doing it. Of course, the opposite is also true. If a supervisor is not happy with a supervisee they too have a responsibility to discuss this with the person. In any case, it does not seem fair to complain about people without giving them the opportunity to do something about it.

Using the 3-Step method to evaluate

The 3-Step method offers structure to an evaluation, irrespective of when it takes place. In other words, I find it just as useful at the end of a session as when it is in the shape of a more formal review of the supervision.

It is important to keep a record of supervision sessions as this will aid continuity of the work and make it easier to provide evidence for its effectiveness. It is also a good idea to keep a record of your evaluations, which can also be structured according to the 3-Step format. This will provide you with evidence regarding the effectiveness of the supervision. It will also help you to track your own development, whether as a supervisor or as a supervisee, as well as the development of the working alliance.

Step 1: What to evaluate?

Both content and process need to be looked at. In other words, we need to ask ourselves:

- What are we working with in supervision and how are we doing that?
- Are we both happy that the content accurately reflects the supervisee's work?
- What do we feel about the way we are working together?

If we keep notes of every session according to the format suggested above, we will have an invaluable source of material to draw on.

During evaluation discussion, useful questions to ask, both of ourselves and of the supervisee, may include:

- What has been happening?
- What has not been happening?
- How do I feel about what has been happening?
- What do I now want to happen in future?

Step 2: How to evaluate?

Evaluation involves not only looking at our own performance and experience, it also means that we need to give each other feedback. While I was on a training course a little while ago, one of the tutors asked, 'What kind of feedback would you like?' I really appreciated that as it gave the recipient control over the process. Some people might say, 'I am feeling rather fragile today, please go easy. I do want to hear where I can improve, but I feel that I can only take it in if it is given to me sensitively.' Other people, who were feeling more robust, might say 'Just give it to me straight!', as they might get frustrated by the softly-softly approach favoured by the first person. If feedback is given in a way that people find uncomfortable, they often do not 'hear' what is said or find it hard to remember.

I find the BOCCS box (Fig. 7.2) a helpful aide memoire to sensitive feedback. BOCCS means that feedback needs to be: balanced, owned, clear, concrete and supportive.

Balance The ability to give balanced feedback is crucial, which is why it is placed right in the centre of the box. Basically it involves giving people a 'feedback sandwich'. This means that you first say what you find positive, then what you would like to be different, followed again by something positive. Many of us have a tendency to focus on what we perceive as shortcomings, rather than on what we are doing well. Framing areas to be worked on within positive feedback helps to put things in perspective.

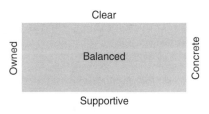

Figure 7.2 The feedback BOCCS box.

Owned   We cannot escape the fact that our feedback is based on our own experience and is therefore subjective. I believe that it is therefore only fair that we own up to that fact. For example, it is more honest to say 'I experienced your saying … as a criticism' rather than 'You are very critical of me.' Owning our own experience also makes it easier for people to take on board what we say; after all, no one can argue with our experience of things. They may say, 'That is not how I experience things,' but they cannot say 'You are not experiencing that.' In my experience, 'owned' feedback can provide an excellent way in which to engage in an honest dialogue.

Clear   It may seem kind to fudge things, but it actually isn't. Clear, unambiguous feedback is much more helpful than feedback that is only half understood. Also, it is good to be brief as too much information may hide or swamp what you are actually trying to say.

Concrete   It is good to link your feedback to concrete examples or events. For example, you may say, 'When you said …' or 'When we were discussing … it felt a bit sticky to me/I felt very supported/criticised,' etc. Just saying, 'I feel supported or criticised' in general is less useful, as people may not understand what it is that you are talking about.

Supportive   Feedback needs to be constructive. In other words, whether we are the supervisor or the supervisee its function is to help us grow and develop and to make the working alliance stronger and (even) more effective. It can be helpful to frame positive comments in terms of 'It would be good if you were to do more of …' Comments regarding behaviours that you would like to be different could be phrased 'I would find it helpful if you were to do less of … ' or 'I would like to encourage you to continue doing …' for positive feedback and 'To develop your ability to … further.' I do not find it particularly helpful to think in terms of negative comments, mistakes or things people do wrong or badly. In general, I prefer to focus on what people do well, and regard what they do not do well as areas that can be developed. Someone's intention to do something, even if they are not quite achieving it, is positive!

Step 3: What have we Now evaluated?

Sometimes feedback, whether it is all positive or whether there are some areas that can be improved on, can be difficult to hold in mind. Once both of you feel that you have come to an end it is therefore useful to take stock of the evaluation by moving on to Step 3. This involves consolidating what has been said by asking each other: 'So what is it that we have heard?'

This then provides an opportunity to check whether both supervisor and supervisee have understood each other's feedback and to clarify anything that is not clear. At this point it may well be useful to make a brief note of the main points.

Once you have understood each other's feedback and have made a record of it, you need to agree on how to go forward by discussing the following:

- What do we want to do Now we have evaluated?
- What do we Now feel about the way we work together?
- What (if anything) do we Now want to change?

At this stage it is important to be as specific as possible and to make a record of this so that both parties are in no doubt as to what has been agreed. This record can be used as a starting point for the next time you evaluate the supervision. For example, both of you may feel that you have been a bit careful with each other and would like to include more challenge in the way you work together. If, the next time you evaluate, both of you are happy with the amount of challenge you receive, this provides clear evidence of the growing effectiveness, both of the working relationship and possibly of the clinical supervision itself.

The evaluation of supervision over time

In this day and age we are often called upon to demonstrate that something is efficient and effective. Regular evaluation of supervision should help to make this process fairly straightforward (van Ooijen 2000:147–150). In any case, it is good practice to evaluate supervision, both at the end of every session and at regular intervals. How frequently you do this may depend on how often you meet. Some people like to evaluate every 3 months, whereas for others once a year seems sufficient. Although some people prefer to evaluate 'ad hoc', I prefer to build it into the working agreement. Not only does this ensure that evaluation happens, it also makes collusion less likely. If you know that you are going to have to say how you are experiencing the supervision, it may be easier to flag up problems than if you have first to create the opportunity to do so.

EVIDENCE

For all of us in the helping professions it is becoming increasingly important to keep a record of what we do so that we can provide evidence for it. Keeping a record of supervision sessions is an obvious way in which such evidence can be acquired. Ideally the notes of a session, whether the supervisor or the supervisee keeps them, should be private and belong to the person who wrote them. However, as will be seen in the next section, they can form the basis for a more public evaluation system with the proviso that what is taken from those notes should be up to the person herself.

Another issue is that, since the Data Protection Act of 1998, individuals now have a right to see any computerised records kept on them, as well as certain categories of manual records. Supervision records could also be requested by the courts in case of a legal dispute between supervisor and supervisee, or when a client sues the agency for which they work (Jenkins 2001:23).

The value of transparency

I feel that if supervisors set out to make the whole issue of record-keeping as transparent as possible, this will go a long way to avoiding problems. Transparency can be achieved in a number of ways. For example, the supervisor can first write the notes and then ask the supervisee to read and sign them if they agree with the content. If there is some discrepancy between the written record and the supervisee's recollection of the session, she can add her version. In any case, discovering such a discrepancy can form a useful basis for an evaluation of how the working alliance is developing. Other possibilities include: the supervisee writing the notes and asking the supervisor to read and sign them; both supervisor and supervisee writing their notes separately but keeping them together in a file; or each writes their own notes and swaps them every few months.

You may well be able to think of yet more ways in which the issue of record-keeping can be made transparent. The advantage of this kind of record-keeping is that there are no mysteries; if there are problems, they will show up as everything is out in the open. It also makes evaluation of the supervision much easier, as both parties know the content of the record (the evidence) on which the evaluation is based.

Using the 3-Step method to write notes

The 3-Step method can be helpful in providing a structure for the writing of notes, both for the supervisor and the supervisee. If, as discussed above, both like to read each other's records, it helps to be familiar with the structure that is being used.

Step 1

- What was the topic (or topics)?
- What were the goals?

Step 2

- How was the focus determined?
- Was the focus mainly 'there and then,' 'here and now' or a balance?
- How was the issue worked with?
- How were skills and methods used?
- How did I experience the working alliance?
- How did I experience the session?
- How did I feel during the session?
- How did the other person feel? (as stated in the evaluation at the end of the session).

Step 3

- What new insights and ideas do I have?
- What was the outcome of the session?
- Were Step1's objectives met?
- What action (if any) was decided upon, and when and how will I carry it out?
- What was useful/not useful?
- What was difficult/not difficult?
- What do I need to think about some more?
- What needs to be discussed or asked about next time?

The method can be used in a flexible way. For example, you may like to take some questions away and substitute them with some of your own that feel more appropriate. Whatever questions you do use, over time the answers written to them will provide a very clear record of how the supervision is progressing.

ENDING THE WORKING ALLIANCE

Ending a relationship is never easy and a supervisory relationship is no different. Many of us may be tempted to fudge the ending. We can do so by, for example, using another commitment as an excuse for not keeping that last appointment, claiming a last minute crisis in work prevents us from coming or whatever. This is particularly likely to happen if the relationship has been uncomfortable and the ending is due to both parties realising that they would rather not continue working together. Uncomfortable though it may be, I think it is really important to have a proper ending. This is because an avoided or fudged ending can lead to any unfinished business spilling over into the next supervisory relationship.

Ideally, endings are already built into the working agreement. I quite like the idea of annual evaluations during which we decide whether we want to continue working together. If we decide that we do, we can either re-affirm our working agreement as it stands, or make such changes as seems appropriate to us both.

If we decide to discontinue our supervisory relationship, we need to work out a plan for doing so. There can be many different reasons for deciding to stop working together, such as:

- One of you is moving away.
- One of you is starting another job, which is making it impossible to continue.
- The supervisee is about to embark on further training and supervision is provided within that.
- Despite having worked hard on your relationship, one or both of you does not feel entirely happy.
- The relationship has become rather too comfortable and you wonder whether it has become collusive.
- You have been working together for quite a few years now and, even though both of you are still happy with the relationship, you both feel that a change may be beneficial and lead to new learning.

USING THE 3-STEP METHOD TO END SUPERVISION

The ending of a supervision relationship needs to be carefully planned in order to prevent unfinished business of this relationship spilling over into the next one. Using the structure provided by the 3-Step method can help ensure that the ending process is given the time and respect it deserves.

Step 1

- What do we want to happen?
- What time frame feels appropriate?
- What will be the last session?

Step 2

- How will we work towards the ending?

Step 3

- What shall we do Now?
- Develop a clear plan: how to work towards an ending; are there any outstanding issues; carry out a final evaluation.

At Step 3 the decisions taken at Step 1 and Step 2 are put together and a clear plan is formulated. In order to learn from their time together both parties need to include a thorough evaluation of the entire time that they have worked together. Particularly if your relationship has been a long one, it is easy to forget how it has changed over time. It can be very illuminating to look back at your records of when you first started to work together. You may be working very harmoniously at the moment and have totally forgotten the sticky patches that you have been through. Looking back may help both of you to consolidate just what you have learnt about each other, about developing a working relationship with someone, about your profession and the way you work and, most of all, about supervision itself. Finally, you may like to write a joint record of your conclusions. I believe this is useful even when the two of you decide that you cannot work together. Somehow it helps to really 'end' something, thus creating a clear space for starting to work with a new person.

CONCLUSION

The focus of this chapter has been on what to do once Step 2, the 'how' of supervision, has been completed. Sometimes this final part of supervision gets overlooked. However, I identified five important elements – learning, action, monitoring, evaluation and evidence – all of which help both the supervisor and the supervisee to keep track of what has been achieved.

I also explained how the 3-Step method may be used for evaluating and writing notes of a supervision session. In the final section I discussed the issue of how to end a supervisory relationship and suggested the 3-Step method as a useful format for managing this process.

Deciding what to do is not always easy, particularly when there appear to be conflicting values and interests at stake. In the next chapter I will therefore focus on such issues and suggest a format for ethical decision-making.

Questions for further reflection

- How do you currently help supervisees to move their practice forward?

- What is your system of evaluation?

- What is your experience of ending supervision, either as a supervisee or as a supervisor?

- Would you have liked the ending to have been different and if so how?

The 3-Step method to ethical decision-making

Are you ruled by your own values or by others' opinions?
(Chakravarty 1997:43)

... do we know the difference between our conscience and our interests? (Wood 2002: 10–11)

This chapter is structured in accordance with the 3-Step method. First, I explain how the 3-Step method can be used as a helpful structure for the making of ethical decisions. Next, I introduce the four ethical principles of beneficence, non-maleficence, justice and autonomy as essential considerations in ethical decision-making. Lastly, I argue how the four principles may be combined with an ethic of care and an awareness of cultural differences.

ETHICAL DECISION-MAKING IS PART OF THE HELPING PROFESSIONAL'S EVERYDAY LIFE

Every situation is unique. Although we may adhere to ethical principles, what we do in practice may vary, depending on the situation. It could be argued that, as helping professionals, everything we do has a direct or indirect impact on the well-being of our clients. Ethical decision-making does not therefore only involve extraordinary situations, but it is part and parcel of our everyday working life. The President of the Royal College of Nursing, Roswyn Hakesley-Brown, states: 'Ethics is, of course, every nurse's business. It's about the everyday decisions – simple and complex – which involve us and our patients' (Hakesley-Brown 2001/2). Working ethically therefore also includes regularly evaluating what we do in supervision and not taking 'collusive rest periods' during which we only pretend to be doing supervision (Bramley 1996:22).

It seems therefore that working ethically means a commitment to 'best practice', particularly as 'the legal and ethical implications of not implementing best practice may be great' (Goss & McLeod 1999). But how do we decide what that best practice is? Every situation is unique and it is therefore not possible to provide easy answers to that question. However, the 3-Step method offers a useful guide to ethical decision-making as follows:

- Step 1: What is the issue?
- Step 2: How do I decide what is the right thing to do?
- Step 3: What will I do Now?

For each step I will offer general guidelines as well as examples of how they can be used in practice. I base my discussion on two main sources: the framework to ethical decision-making offered by Bond (2000) and the complementary approach of an 'ethic of care' (Benner & Wrubel 1989, Noddings 1986, Taylor 1995, Watson 1988).

STEP 1: WHAT IS THE ISSUE?

We need to be clear on what the issue or problem is as well as to whom it belongs. For example, a supervisee was working with a single woman who was tempted to become involved with a married man. The supervisee was happily married herself and felt strongly that extramarital affairs were wrong and likely to cause nothing but grief to all concerned. 'I consider it my ethical duty to advise her against it,' she said, 'as it is not fair on the man's wife. But I am not supposed to give advice am I? I just don't know what to do.'

 THINKING POINT

What do you think the issue is here?

Actually, there are two issues: first, what should the supervisee do? And second, what should the client do? There is often more than one issue involved, which can lead to confusion. A useful question to ask is therefore 'Whose issue is it?' (Bond 2000). It seems clear that what the client should do is her issue and not that of the practitioner. Having identified that the decision whether or not to become involved with a married man is for the client to decide, the practitioner was still unclear how to continue working with the client. 'Oh,' she said, 'I can see that I cannot make decisions for people, after all, it is her life and you are right, I cannot really be sure that it will not work out for her. Maybe his marriage is on the rocks, maybe he will even marry her, who knows.' The above is an example of issue confusion. Having unpacked it a bit it is clear that the ethical decision to be made here is not up to the practitioner, but up to the client. However, if the client's proposed action is against the law, or involves the safety of children, the situation becomes more complex and may need further deliberation.

If the dilemma looks more complex and may be the practitioner's issue, there are a number of useful points to consider:

- What is the legal position on what is happening?
- What are the people concerned (including the practitioner) entitled to by law?
- What actions (if any) are the people concerned (including the practitioner) legally obliged to take?

STEP 2: HOW DO I DECIDE WHAT IS THE RIGHT THING TO DO?

Once you, as the supervisor, have clarified that the issue does involve either you yourself and/or the practitioner and you have checked that there are no legal complications, the question 'How do I decide what is right?' or 'How do I help the supervisee to decide what is right?' needs to be addressed. For example, imagine that while you are supervising a newly qualified practitioner you become concerned by her standard of work. Even though she is no longer a novice, she does not appear to be making any progress and is not working to the standard that could reasonably be expected. Although you have bent over backwards to facilitate her development, it is as if all your efforts are poured into a leaky pot. During the sessions you have with her she appears to be making progress, but when you next see her it as if the previous session never took place. However, the supervisee always gives a professional impression and can talk volubly and articulately. You therefore feel that you may be the only person who is noticing that she is not delivering the 'best practice' expected of her.

THINKING POINT

How would you decide what to do?

In making any ethical decision there are four main principles that need to be looked at:

1. Beneficence: what will achieve the greatest good?
2. Non-maleficence: what will cause the least harm?
3. Justice: what will be fairest?
4. Respect for autonomy: what maximises the opportunities for everyone involved to implement their choices?

Let's look at each one in turn.

BENEFICENCE/NON-MALEFICENCE

For both beneficence and non-maleficence we need to ask 'Who do we mean when we talk about good or harm?'

THINKING POINT

Who do you think any positive good or harm applies to?

The players in this example are the supervisee, her clients and the employing organisation. What is good for one is not necessarily good for the other. For example, the supervisee may regard being allowed to continue as normal as 'good' for her and unlikely to cause her harm. However, her poor standard of practice is already likely to affect her clients adversely and could, if it remains unchecked, lead to serious consequences. If that happens, the organisation will be harmed too, both in terms of its reputation and possibly also financially. The people managing the supervisee are also likely to be harmed as they may be held responsible. But lastly, you, the supervisor, are likely to be harmed as it is you who has the task of monitoring her work. In this case non-action is likely to lead to harm for all concerned. Even the supervisee herself may be harmed if, at some stage, she makes a gross error and is charged with misconduct or negligence. However, the harm that has to have the greatest weight is the actual and possible harm done to the client. Even if the client is the only one harmed by non-action and it is better for all other parties to do nothing, the client's welfare is paramount. This is because all of us in the helping professions have a 'duty of care'; it is what we are about and it is implicit in any practitioner–client interaction. Our duty of care to our clients implies our clients' right to that care.

Supervisors need to keep an eye out for the possibility of harm being done to clients, although most of the time this is likely to be unintentional rather than deliberate. Ethical issues often come to the notice of the supervisor accidentally. It is not unusual for supervisees to bring an issue about which they are not sure and are feeling vaguely uncomfortable (Bramley 1996:82). Sometimes this means that the principle of 'do no harm' is involved.

For example, as far as the practice of counselling is concerned, there is the possibility of the counsellor unwittingly injuring a client by making an ill-timed comment or interpretation. Occasionally such a comment may be motivated by an unconscious (and therefore unrecognised) part of the counsellor's personality. Even if the interpretation is technically correct, it can be experienced as abusive if it is made clumsily, ill-timed, or perhaps motivated by an unconscious desire in the counsellor rather than for the client's benefit (Bramley 1996:83). It is the counselling supervisor's task to watch out for such events, as the counsellor herself may not be aware of what is happening. This is also one of the reasons why the British Association for Counselling and Psychotherapy advocates that counsellors undergo counselling or therapy themselves, and many counselling courses insist on people receiving personal therapy throughout their training. The more aware the counsellor becomes of her own processes the less likely it is that she will unconsciously act out something with a client, although there can never be a guarantee that this will not happen.

Various books have been written by clients who feel they were damaged by their counsellor or therapist (Heyward 1994).

Whereas I do not wish to comment here on these examples, I know from experience how painful it can be (for the worker as well as the client) when a client feels that you are being abusive. Some years ago a client whom I had been seeing for quite a long time was furious with me about something I had said in the previous session. I felt confused, as there appeared to be quite a mismatch between what he had heard and what I remembered myself actually saying. However, the client remained adamant in sticking to his version. Although there was clearly a transference issue, I felt uneasy and took it to supervision. When we reflected on the last few sessions, it became clear that, although my interpretation appeared accurate, the client was not yet ready to receive it. My supervisor felt that as my work with this client had been careful up to this point, the clumsy timing seemed out of character and indicative of possible unconscious motivation. Subsequent exploration in both supervision and my personal therapy provided further clarity, which helped me to continue working with the client. However, it was a salutary experience for me, from which I learnt that harm can be done unwittingly and that it is therefore important to stay vigilant and continue to be open to our own processes and personal development. 'It is not unethical to have bad feelings about a patient. It is unethical not to examine them' (Bramley 1996:105). Helping supervisees to become aware of any negative feelings makes it less likely that they will act them out and thus injure the client.

JUSTICE: WHAT WILL BE FAIREST?

Here we have to ensure that justice is done by all equally. For example, it might seem easiest for the organisation to sack the supervisee and employ a more skilled person instead. This would be good for the clients as well as the organisation, but it would be unfair to the supervisee. She would be completely in her rights to sue for 'unfair' dismissal, as she had not been involved in any discussions in how to solve the problem.

RESPECT FOR AUTONOMY

This means that every person should be treated with equal respect. It also means that each person is an autonomous individual who has the right to make her own decisions regarding her own life. With regard to the earlier example, respect for autonomy means that it is up to the client and not the practitioner to decide whether or not to start an affair with a married man. Of course this does not mean that it cannot be talked about, but respect for autonomy means not forcing our judgements on other people.

Like good, harm and justice, autonomy also applies to everyone involved. Regarding the issue of the incompetent supervisee, respect for autonomy may mean informing her of the dilemma, so that she can make a choice as to what to do. Autonomy also applies to the other players; all need to be aware in order to make a choice. For example, if the supervisee were to put pressure on the supervisor to turn a blind eye, that would be in violation of the supervisor's autonomy.

Respect for autonomy also means not going beyond the limits of your competence, either as a practitioner or as a supervisor. If you are inexperienced as a supervisor, being honest about it will honour your supervisees' autonomy and allow them to make up their minds whether or not to work with you. Being honest will also allow you and your supervisees to learn and grow together. Supervisees may well prefer a novice supervisor, as they are likely to be perceived as less threatening. Also, it is not necessarily the case that the more experienced supervisor is also the better one.

As far as clients are concerned, if you are working in the mental health field, respect for their autonomy means enlisting their healthy self, by which I mean the adult or healthy part of the person's personality. This is the part that can look at himself and his past objectively; it is also likely to be that part of his personality that prompted him to seek help and that needs to be engaged with in order to create a therapeutic alliance. Supervisors need to monitor supervisees' work in order to ensure that respect for autonomy is practised; they also need to demonstrate it in their own work. In practice, this includes finding out physical and practical aspects of the supervisee's work. For counsellors and other professionals this may mean checking out the boundaries of their work, such as a safe place and set times (as modelled by the clinical supervision itself) (Bramley 1996:93).

Waiting time is in itself an ethical issue. In private counselling or therapy, sticking to pre-arranged times is regarded as sacrosanct and part of providing a safe container for the client within which their anxiety and concerns can be looked at. I feel that in other therapy services, such as medical, nursing and the professions allied to medicine, such safety may be equally important.

Picture the following: you have been investigated for a lump in your breast or testes and this morning you have a 9.30 appointment with the doctor to hear the result. Now imagine that 9.30 comes and goes – wouldn't you get restless? I bet that the longer you have to wait, the more nervous you will become. In fact, by the time you get to see the doctor you may be so worked up that it becomes difficult to take in what is being said to you. Clearly the principles of 'do no harm' and 'do good' are not being adhered to here. An ethic of care, which is a stance or frame of mind, makes it possible to work within the four principles without losing sight of the client. Without such an ethic of care it is easy to forget the client as other, often organisational, issues seem to predominate. (This will be discussed in more detail later in the chapter.)

Another effect of being kept waiting, particularly if this is regarded as the norm, is to feel unvalued, not important. Being given a hospital appointment for 9.30 and then being kept waiting for up to 2 hours (as has happened to me on quite a few occasions) implies that my time is not important. Clearly, I have nothing better to do than wait for the doctor, whose time, of course, is more important than anyone else's. As I have no influence in the matter the principle of autonomy, 'my autonomy' is violated; also it implies a lack of respect.

It is possible, even for the most dedicated professionals, to become complacent regarding this and other issues. To keep people waiting may become so much part of the norm that it is seen as a given, with the result that people are kept waiting even when it is not really necessary. For example, a case conference may be started late, then finish late, so that everyone is late for their next appointment, and so on.

I feel it is within the normative function of supervision to challenge complacency and to help the supervisee look at all aspects of their practice with fresh eyes ('super' vision). Although I realise that there are things the supervisee really has no control over, often people are not as powerless as they believe.

CULTURAL DIFFERENCES

Each one of us sees the world through the window of his thoughts. (Chakravarty 1997:12)

At this point I want to make two more points about Step 2. Although the four principles are very useful, it should not be forgotten that they constitute a Western ethic and that other cultures may look at things differently. What we decide as causing harm, or doing good, for example, may be seen differently by a person from a non-Western background. Also, our emphasis on autonomy and individuality is not necessarily shared by other cultures, where the family or the group may be regarded as all-important, and where decision-making may not be just up to the individual.

Our society is becoming more and more multicultural and it is therefore important that we stay open to the different ways the world can be perceived. Regarding supervision, various cultural combinations may occur, such as:

- Culturally dominant supervisor – different culture supervisee – culturally dominant client.
- Culturally dominant supervisor – culturally dominant supervisee – different culture client.
- Different culture supervisor – culturally dominant supervisee – culturally dominant client, and so on.

Take, for example, the case of a white supervisor supervising a white supervisee, who is working with an Asian man. There is probably a limit to the extent that we can really understand the problems of an Asian man in his relations with his family.

Differences in culture are not always obvious and can therefore easily be overlooked. In my own case, whereas I am white, my culture of origin is not English. However, I have been in the UK for a long time and therefore assumed until fairly recently that it was not really relevant. Certainly, within a professional context, it was usually the last thing on my mind, so I assumed this to be the same for other people who are different, whether by sexuality, culture, class, race or whatever. Because of various experiences I now know just how much culture colours what we experience and how easy it is for misunderstandings to occur. What I have learnt is that we can never assume that we know how someone else is experiencing the world, or that others will understand my experience.

As we are all influenced both by the culture in which we grew up and the one in which we find ourselves, the way in which we look at the world in general, and at ethical issues in particular, may vary. What seems important to me is to recognise this fact, to talk openly about this with supervisees, and to encourage them to do the same with their clients. A good beginning may be 'As a white woman I experience this as … but I am aware that it may be very different for you. Can you tell me how you experience it?' This may then become a dialogue in which the two of you can talk openly and honestly about your differences in order to get a sense of the other's point of view.

AN ETHIC OF CARE

The second point I want to make is that it is useful to see the four principles within an overall framework of an ethic of care (see Fig. 8.1). This is because a potential problem with principles such as beneficence and non-maleficence is that what is regarded as good or bad depends on who is doing the judging. Professionals may feel that they know what is good for a client better than the client herself, which is, of course, a violation of the principle of autonomy. So it is useful to check the principles out against each other. An ethic of care forms another useful check. In a way, the four principles approach may be seen as a 'masculine' way of ethical decision-making, with an ethic of care providing a 'feminine' counter-balance. There can often be a clear gender difference in the way men and women approach ethical issues, with men employing detached, rational hierarchical forms of reasoning based on principles (Noddings 1986:5). Women, on the other hand, tend to find this type of reasoning abstract and meaningless and prefer to see the issue in its context and in terms of the relevant relationships.

It has been suggested that some situations, such as economic deprivation, affect men and women in similar ways, leading to

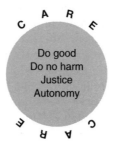

Care=what does all
this look like from inside?

Figure 8.1 The four principles of ethical decision-making within a framework of an ethic of care.

convergence in their moral views (Stack in Larrabee 1993). Rather than continuing to talk about gender differences, real or otherwise, it would seem useful to develop a synthesis in terms of 'what kind of morality is desirable' for men as well as for women. A reasonable feminist goal might therefore be to enable women as well as men to choose when it is appropriate to be concerned with abstract issues and when with caring and relatedness (Luria 1993). Although different, the concepts of care and justice are not actually incompatible, as treating someone justly is likely to imply caring about that person (Friedman 1987 cited by Larrabee 1993).

Rationality and emotion do not need to be seen in opposition. I see both as subsidiary to the larger concept of care (Watson 1988). Care does not just involve being nice to people, it also involves knowledge and judgement resulting in concrete acts and outcomes. Caring therefore involves a commitment to excellence, expertise and best practice and a furthering of knowledge by research as well as theoretical development. In other words, a commitment to care as an ethical ideal incorporates a striving for excellence in order to get the most desirable outcomes for the people being cared for (Benner & Wrubel 1989, Watson 1988).

Thus, caring is always to be understood in context, technical proficiency being appropriate in one situation, emotional support in another, cure being dependent upon care and caring practices. For example, people whose disease has caused their quality of life to be apparently severely reduced, may make sense of things not in terms of what they have lost or can no longer do, but in terms of what is still possible. Life goes on, even for the terminally ill (Benner & Wrubel 1989:xi). In this context, I remember a woman, emaciated and bedridden with cancer, whose main concern was to visit her solicitor in person to sort out her affairs for the benefit of her dependants. The nurse looking after her was able to 'receive' her and realise the meaning of this visit and enabled the patient to do so with a fair amount of organisation, time and resources. From a curing point of view, the visit was neither necessary nor perhaps advisable; from a caring perspective it was crucial. It was the appropriate ethical decision.

THE IMPORTANCE OF NOW

Benner and Wrubel's position is useful in that they stress the importance of the present. Care is therefore securely grounded in the present; it has a 'dynamic quality' (Pirsig 1978) as it is the present experience that matters. Benner and Wrubel point out that caring is a 'good in itself'. They regard a traditional, paternalistic, curing view – according to which 'good' is defined by the professional rather than the patient – as mistaken and illogical. Only if the practitioner and client share their phenomenological field and common humanity, and the one caring is in tune with the cared for, will the notion of what is 'good' be agreed and will the principle of beneficence be accorded its true status.

Another matter for consideration is that our Western values such as autonomy or privacy are not necessarily shared by other cultures, whereas care and being cared for are valued universally. Benner & Wrubel (1989) regard the, sometimes extreme, individualism of Western culture and the association of caring with the role of women as damaging, in that it perpetuates a split, dualistic view of individuals as well as of society. Devaluing care leads to an overemphasis on so-called curing techniques which are becoming increasingly technological. In this light it is possible to imagine a patient wired up to a lot of technological apparatus which is continuously being monitored, with the person of the patient not really being acknowledged and certainly not feeling cared for.

> *It's not what you do that counts, it's what you are.*
> (Kugler 1995:33)

The above quote is as relevant to the worker as it is to the supervisor. When I reflect on my work and my experiences, it seems to me, and perhaps also to you, that everything I do and choose to get involved with is part of a bigger picture. Whatever I do and how I do it reflects where I am at that particular moment – it reflects my own personal development.

Caring essentially involves relationships and thus necessitates looking at things through the eyes both of the practitioner and of the client. This means that the supervisee needs to be given the opportunity to show off what she is doing well and receive praise for that, as well as being able to talk about the problems she is encountering (Bramley 1996:16). Caring also implies action, a wanting to reduce any suffering or pain on the part of the one being cared for. In order to care for others in this way we need to have a sense of what kind of things give pain and pleasure to ourselves. An ethic of care therefore implies a commitment to self-knowledge and self-awareness. To work truly ethically we cannot stop working on our own growth and development, whether in the form of personal counselling, therapy or whatever means seems appropriate. Ethical supervision therefore includes facilitating such growth and development in the supervisee (Bramley 1996:17).

My own take on an ethic of care is that it involves being prepared to get a real sense of what another person experiences, to 'enter their phenomenological field', to attempt to see the world through their eyes (Benner & Wrubel 1989, Noddings 1986). Such an ethic seems also pertinent to intercultural relationships as discussed above. This is because I cannot know what your experience is without being prepared to really listen (with body and soul) to what you are telling me. This kind of listening is not easy and we may bump into our defences and filters. But as long as we notice the bump, recognise the defence and are prepared to look at it and perhaps set it aside for the moment, we have a chance of really 'being with' the other person.

EXAMPLE: THE VALUE OF PERSONAL EXPERIENCE

A few years ago I experienced what it was like to be at the other side of the helping professions when I was admitted to hospital. It was nothing serious, just some minor surgery, which meant that I only needed to be an inpatient for 3 days. However, the experience was quite disorienting and 2 months after the event I wrote in my reflective journal that I had not quite recovered from it and was tempted to deny that anything had really happened. And yet my experience had not been especially bad. Things were fairly uneventful and the staff were not unpleasant. And yet I found myself pondering on what it means to be part of a helping and caring profession. I asked myself 'What is it about?' and 'What should it be about?' What my experience brought home to me was that there are two entirely different worlds: the world of the patients (clients or users) and the world of the professionals.

I was surprised just how the fact of being in hospital affected me. Suddenly my freedom of movement was severely restricted and most of my activities were under the gaze of others. I was lucky to be given a private room to which I could retreat, but even so felt very visible, as the door was usually open. There were all kinds of things I could not do, which I normally take for granted, such as making myself a coffee or picking up the phone. In fact, I could not even have a glass of water unless I was given a special jug, as all taps had a notice saying 'not for drinking'. Although I realise that part of the way I felt was due to the effect of the anaesthetic, I don't think that this was the whole story. Somehow my head felt like cottonwool, simply from being in the hospital ward environment 24 hours a day. This cottonwool feeling disappeared miraculously once I was discharged. As soon as I got home I was able to think again, and what a relief that was. But most of all, I felt a normal human being again, a person, entitled to being treated as such. Somehow things felt very different when I was a patient; the normal rules of social conduct did not necessarily seem to apply.

I now value this experience as it taught me just how differently we experience the world when we are in a position other than the one we are used to. I knew hospitals well as I had worked in them for many years, so, if the experience had such a profound effect on me, how much more must people be affected who have no such experience. As far as supervision is concerned, I like to encourage supervisees to really engage in a dialogue with their clients in order to get a sense of what their experience is like. Wouldn't it be great if it was part of normal practice, for every patient, client or user, to have someone really interested in them and their experience. It seems to me that this would be very healing. Similarly, it is important for the supervisor to be committed to understanding what the supervision experience is like for the supervisee. What is needed is a commitment to growth and a willingness to be open and honest. It is also good for supervisors as well as supervisees not to be afraid to be vulnerable at times or to admit to being wrong.

ONLY CONNECT

No-one is an island, each one of us is connected to everyone else, but each of us needs one person to receive a special focus from, to be 'seen'. In other words, we need somehow to convey to clients as well as supervisees 'I see what is happening to you, really see it.' How often do we really see the people we call patients or clients? How often do we really let ourselves see or feel what is happening? What the world is like for that person? To do that we have to step outside our own frame of reference and come on the inside, alongside the patient. The world will seem a different place. We may not even recognise the care environment. But, in order to really be the practitioner that we can be, we must, perhaps paradoxically, step out of our professional world and into the one of the client.

ENTERING THE WORLD OF THE CLIENT

There are various techniques that can help us to enter the world of our clients. In the actual situation there is no substitute for genuine dialogue (Hycner & Jacobs 1995). In supervision it is often very useful to ask the supervisee briefly to take the role of the client, with the supervisor playing the supervisee. This often leads to a shift in the supervisee's view of the situation. Sometimes it is helpful to have the supervisor playing the client, with the supervisee playing herself. If other people are involved in the ethical dilemma it may also be useful to role-play their positions.

During the role-play each ethical principle can be examined in turn in order to find out how the situation impacts on the person being played.

Other techniques may involve asking the supervisee to imagine that they are their client and to 'rapid write' a page or so from that position (rapid writing was discussed in Chapter 4). Visualisation can also be helpful. Here the supervisee is asked to close her eyes while the supervisor talks her through the situation.

STEP 3: WHAT NOW?

Having unpacked the situation by looking at how all players are affected in terms of the four principles, it becomes necessary to try and make a decision. At this point it is useful to brainstorm all possible courses of action and work out which one:

- Creates the most good, particularly for the client.
- Does the least harm, particularly for the client.
- Treats everyone fairly.
- Respects everyone's autonomy.

Having selected your preferred course of action Bond (2000) suggests asking yourself the following questions:

- Could I recommend this action to others?
- If I heard about someone who had done what I propose to do, would I condone it?

- Could I explain my action to my colleagues/supervisor/other practitioners?
- Would I be happy to have my action scrutinised?
- Would I do the same for any client?
- Would I do the same if the supervisee/client was a famous person?

If the answer to any of these six questions is 'No', there may be something wrong with your proposed action, and you may need to think again (Bond 2000).

Having carried out the action, it is also useful to evaluate the outcome in order to find out:

- Was it the right thing?
- If not, what have I learnt from it?
- How might I do it differently in the future?

With regard to the incompetent supervisee, the supervisor decided to talk about it openly with the supervisee. It transpired that the supervisee felt overwhelmed by problems in her personal life. She agreed to talk to her organisation herself and gave permission for the organisation to contact the supervisor if they wanted more information. After talking with her manager, the supervisee decided to take a year out, during which her personal problems would hopefully be resolved and she would decide whether or not to continue in that particular chosen profession. When the supervisor evaluated the outcome, she felt that her action had been appropriate, but she resolved to act much earlier if a similar situation arose in the future in order to minimise any possible harm to clients.

CONCLUSION

In this chapter I discussed in some detail how the 3-Step method can be used to help supervisees work ethically. I have argued that there is more to ethics than the occasional dilemma and that ethics involves everything we do as a helping professional. The four ethical principles were suggested as a useful guide to ethical decision-making if used in conjunction with an ethic of care. I suggest that in the case of ethical dilemmas it can be helpful for the supervisee to take the role of each player in the scenario in turn in order to get a sense of how the four principles impact on each individual. The greater understanding thus gained will then hopefully facilitate the supervisee to make a decision that maximises the good for the client and minimises harm done to others.

Questions for further reflection

- Take some time to reflect on your last working day. What ethical decisions have you made? With hindsight, can you say which principles were involved? How did you make your decision?

- Look at the issue again in light of the discussion in this chapter. Would you change anything?

9

Applying the 3-Step method to group supervision

Potentially, the group is the supervisor. As a supervisor it contains not only the resources of supervisor and each group member, but, in embryo, the rich creativity of a complex living group system. (Proctor 2000:17)

As the way in which a group is set up will greatly influence its success, I first discuss the nature of group development and some of the associated dynamics. Next I introduce the 3-Step method as a useful vehicle for the consideration of some important questions to the formation of a group's working agreement, followed by a range of useful tools and techniques for the actual 'doing' of the supervision. Lastly, I discuss the importance of bringing unconscious processes into the open, both for the 'task' and for the 'maintenance' of a supervision group.

DEVELOPMENT OF A SUPERVISION GROUP

WHY CHOOSE GROUP SUPERVISION?

Many people, myself included, like to be part of a supervision group in addition to their individual supervision arrangements. Others choose to be members of a group in preference to supervision that is one-to-one. Whichever form you choose will depend not only on the kind of work you do, but also on your feelings about groups in general. Like most things, there are advantages and disadvantages to group supervision (van Ooijen 2000:32–34). Before deciding to join a group it may therefore be useful to ask yourself what your reasons are for doing so and to be clear on what you want from a group that you do not get from one-to-one supervision.

STAGES IN THE LIFE OF A GROUP

Nearly 40 years ago Tuckman discovered that there are definite stages in the life of a group (Tuckman 1965). I have found Tuckman's work very useful in helping to explain some of my experiences with groups. In total there are five stages: forming, storming, norming, performing and adjourning.

The forming stage

In this stage people have only just got together. Although some people may have met each other before, the group as a whole is a new one. People tend to interact in the formal, polite way that is characteristic in communications with strangers. As the group does not yet have an identity of its own, people tend to look to a leader for clues regarding what is or is not acceptable. If the potential supervision group is facilitated, the group supervisor will fulfil this role. In an unfacilitated group it is likely that one person may, for the time being at any rate, function as an unofficial leader. Before the group can start to work it is therefore important that time is spent on getting to know each other. Whatever group we join, we tend to subtly assess other people in order to see how similar or different they are to us. At this stage we may begin to develop preferences for some people rather than others, which means that, in a large group, various alliances and subgroups may begin to form. Also people tend to opt for safety rather than conflict, which is reflected in the discussions that take place.

The storming stage

Here people tend to begin to organise themselves for the task in hand, which inevitably brings with it conflict and competition. The larger the group, the less likely it is that everyone will agree on everything and compromise is therefore needed if the group is going to function effectively. In order to feel safe there may be an increased emphasis on developing a tight structure and rules of conduct. This can be an uncomfortable stage, with some people holding the fort while others feel too threatened to say very much. Eventually though, the group needs to develop in such a way as to help everyone to feel safe enough to participate equally. In order to move on to the next stage, people need to listen to each other, which will help the group to move away from competition and conflict to the solving of problems.

The norming stage

Here the group has formed into a cohesive unit. All members are actively involved in maintaining the group and solving any problems. Subgroups and cliques tend to dissolve, so the group feels much closer. People often feel relieved that the earlier conflict has been resolved and have a sense of belonging. The group is now effectively accomplishing the task for which it was formed. There is a great deal of sharing thoughts, feelings and ideas, as well as the giving of feedback to each other. This stage is often very enjoyable, but has a possible drawback of people wanting to maintain the status quo and therefore resisting any further change.

The performing stage

A transcending of the resistance to change is essential to this stage and not all groups are able to reach it. This is a dynamic stage, which is characterised by true interdependence. This means that there are no fixed ways in which people behave as roles adjust according to the needs, both of the group and of the individuals within it. Regarding the task, productivity is high. People are not afraid to experiment and take risks, as they know that they will be supported. There is a strong sense of group identity and loyalty and the morale of the group is high.

The adjourning stage

If a group needs to be discontinued, it is important to do so in a planned and careful way. Particularly if the group functioned really well, its dissolution means a loss to the people concerned, which needs to be recognised. It is helpful for members to have the opportunity to express to each other their appreciation and to be able to take leave of each other in a way that honours the group as well as each other.

ROLES AND BEHAVIOURS

Particularly during the first two stages, people tend to adopt specific roles and exhibit certain behaviours. Whichever role or behaviour is chosen will to some extent depend on one's previous experience of groups.

 THINKING POINT

At this point it may be good to stop reading. Imagine that you are about to be involved in the setting up of a supervision group. How would you answer the following questions?

Roles
- What roles are possible in this group?
- Which roles are desirable and which undesirable?
- What kind of role do I tend to take and how do I feel about that?
- What would I like to do differently?
- What different role would I like to take?
- What help would I like from other group members?

Behaviours
- What kind of behaviours have I experienced in a group?
- Which ones would I like to see more of in this group?
- Which ones would I like to see less of in this group?

SETTING UP A SUPERVISION GROUP

A supervision group is a special kind of group, which may be expected to function effectively almost immediately. However, as is clear from the above discussion on the development of groups, all groups go through a series of stages before they become really effective. In order to be able to work 'well enough' reasonably quickly, it is useful for members to be aware of these stages as it can help understand what is happening and lessen any potentially destructive behaviours. In other words, I am talking about making the process of group development conscious. The 3-Step method can be helpful in this – each step comprising an essential stage in the development of a working agreement.

STEP 1: THE 'WHAT' OF A WORKING AGREEMENT

This step concerns the development of the structure within which the supervision will take place.

Questions to address

- What kind of a group is this?
- What is the professional background of group members?
- What existing links already exist between individual group members?
- What other information do we want to gain about each other?
- What kind of group do we want?
- What is the function of the group? Its purpose? Its task?
- What are individual members' expectations? Wants? Don't wants? Learning styles?
- What roles and behaviours do individual members tend to adopt in groups?
- What are the dynamics that could surface?
- What model do we want to adopt?
- What methods do we want to use?
- What skills do individual members want to develop?
- What ground rules need to be put in place regarding: practicalities (where to meet, when, how long for, how often), attendance, cancellations?
- What else do we need to consider?

If a supervision group consists of members of the same team there are additional issues that need to be looked at relating to authority, seniority and accountability. As I discuss in Chapter 10, team supervision can be good for team development, but it can also be difficult, as sooner or later problems of the larger organisation will get played out in the group. A psychodynamic model of working, such as the one discussed in the final section of this chapter, may be helpful in such a case.

Whatever the background of its members, though, as far as the group is concerned there is always a certain amount of interdependence. Mutual respect is therefore crucial, with every member taking responsibility for their own behaviour. This is especially important in a peer-led group. This means that if a group is not functioning well through defensive behaviour, personality clashes or other problems, each member is equally responsibile for bringing this out into the open.

In practice, setting up a group is not fundamentally different to starting individual supervision. In whatever way potential group members have come together, there is a need to get to know each other. This will include finding out about each other's professional background. If some people already know each other in some other capacity it is good to bring this out in the open and discuss whether it could militate against the cohesiveness of the group or whether there might be issues of safety or confidentiality.

Other issues that need to be discussed and agreed concern the frequency of meetings, the length of the sessions and where the supervision will take place. The consistency of attendance that the group requires also needs to be clear, as well as what policy people want to adopt regarding cancellations, whether the group is closed or open and what the procedure should be for leaving the group, or for the selection of new members.

STEP 2: THE 'HOW' OF A WORKING AGREEMENT

Having explored the potential structure of the group, the actual process also needs to be discussed. Here, it is useful to consider the four main styles of supervision in groups that have been identified (Proctor 2000:38).

Authoritative   This is basically one-to-one supervision with other group members acting as an audience. This style is useful for those new to group supervision, or as a demonstration of models, tools or methods that group members may be unfamiliar with.

Participative   The supervisor is in charge of the supervision, but also invites group members' participation. Here members are beginning to learn how to supervise.

Cooperative   Here the supervisor acts as a facilitator rather than as a group leader. All members take responsibility for what they want from the group and are actively involved in supervising each other.

Peer group   In a peer group there is no permanent supervisor. Group members may either share overall responsibility or take turns to take the role of facilitator.

A peer group can work very well, particularly if people are experienced in group supervision. It is important, however, to develop and stick to a clear structure as shared responsibility could lead to no responsibility being taken. Peer groups can on occasion resemble a school playground with all kinds of games being played. Some of the problems that may occur are:

- Not everyone participates equally: shyer members may hide, others may 'free load'.
- The group is competitive, everyone wanting to be the 'best' professional, the person with the greatest insight, or the one who has read the latest books and so on.
- The group may collude in not challenging each other (mutual admiration society).
- Time is wasted in small talk.
- People shy away from deeper reflection, preferring to ask for and offer advice.
- The group becomes negative and colludes in feeling powerless.
- One person may be singled out to act as scapegoat.
- The group may become pre-occupied with its own dynamics rather than focusing on the actual supervision (van Ooijen 2000:33).

Questions to address

- How are we going to work together?
- How will we ensure a safe environment?
- How will we know whether the group is functioning well?
- How will we work with group dynamics, particularly if things get difficult?

- How will we know when the group is not fulfilling its potential?
- How will we ensure that everyone's needs get met?
- How will we ensure that everyone's learning styles are accommodated?
- How will we ensure equal participation?
- How will we accommodate differences in professional background or theoretical orientation?
- How will we resolve ethical problems?
- How will we help each other develop facilitation skills?
- How will we choose:
  —Who facilitates?
  —The style of facilitation?
  —The model to be used?
  —Methods to be used?
  —How we use the time?
  —Who is supervised?

This may seem like a long list of questions, but in practice I find that people do not necessarily need an enormously long time to discuss them. I do think, though, that at least flagging them up and noting down what is decided in the working agreement can prevent problems later. In any case, as with one-to-one supervision, the working agreement can be revised and amended whenever all participants feel the need to do so. As far as the role of facilitator is concerned, I would see my role as helping the group to grow and develop in such a way that I will eventually become superfluous.

STEP 3: THE 'WHAT NOW' STEP TO A WORKING AGREEMENT

The discussions that took place under Steps 1 and 2 now need to be firmed up into actual decisions in order to produce a working document. I call it a working agreement rather than a contract, as it is a good idea to agree to take another look at it after three or four sessions. No matter how thorough the discussion has been, not every eventuality can be predicted and some issues may only occur once people start working together. It is therefore advisable to retain some flexibility and not to tie things down too early. Also, depending on the context in which the supervision group is set up, there may be organisational constraints and requirements that need to be considered. In such cases, a two- or three-way contract may need to be developed (group and organisation or facilitator, group and organisation).

Questions to address

- What have we decided on each point?
- What rules do all accept?
- What is the time-span of this agreement?
- What working agreement have we come up with?

USE OF THE 3-STEP METHOD FOR WORKING IN A GROUP

The 3-Step method may be used to structure a group supervision session. The three main questions to be addressed in this respect are:

- What shall we do first?
- Who will be the supervisee?
- What is the issue?

STEP 1: THE 'WHAT' STEP
What shall we do first?

It is a good idea to set aside a set amount of time for a check-in. Unless people work together they may not have seen each other since the last supervision session and want to exchange some social information. Also, it can be helpful to get a sense of how everyone is feeling before starting.

Who will be the supervisee?

A variety of methods may be used to choose who will be the supervisee or supervisees in a session:

- Everyone is expected to work at every session, so the time is always divided equally between the members present.
- Not everyone works every time; instead, people take turns to be supervisee. How many people can take the role of super- visee during any one session will depend on the size of the group as well as how long it meets. So it may work out that every member gets a turn every two or three sessions.
- A round robin: every member says whether or not they want to work. Then the time can either be divided equally or people can say how much time they need.
- Bidding for time. This is a variation of the round robin method. It may be that too many people want to work, causing the avail- able time per individual to be too short for it to be useful. People may 'bid', using their need for supervision or the inter- est of the topic or the general usefulness of the issue, for other members as the currency, so to speak.

With all methods, the order in which people take the role of super- visee also needs to be negotiated. Care needs to be taken with the round robin and bidding for time methods so that, over time, everyone takes an equal part. Thus it may be helpful for some kind of group record to be kept. If this is not done there is the dan- ger that some people may get a great deal of attention, with others feeling that they are missing out. Also, the people who do not often act as supervisee may be resented by other members. They may be seen as withholding something, or acting superior, making other members feel less safe.

What is the issue?

Once the supervisees have been identified, the actual process is similar to one-to-one supervision in that they need to be helped to first of all be clear about the focus and to identify what it is they want to get out of the session (see Chapter 3).

STEP 2: THE 'HOW' STEP

The actual process of supervision can feel very different to indi- vidual work. Whether there is a regular facilitator or whether members of the group take turns to facilitate a session, the actual style adopted needs to be negotiated. Particularly in peer group supervision the fourth style identified by Proctor (2000) tends to be adopted, with people participating as and when they want to. This needs to be well facilitated or the supervisee may feel overwhelmed and unable to make use of people's input. Particularly when a group is new it may be useful to process members' input via the facilitator. Not only will this ensure that the supervisee is not asked to process too much at once, it can also help ensure that all members are helped to take an equal part in making supervisory comments.

In addition to negotiating the style to be used, it is also helpful to agree a model or method. There are a number of models, tools and techniques that lend themselves particularly well to supervision in a group. Potentially the group is a rich resource, not only of knowledge and experience, but also of exploring issues in ways that are not possible with only two people.

STEP 3: 'WHAT NOW?'

There are two elements to Step 3: the identification of vicarious learning – i.e. the learning that has taken place for the group members other than the supervisee; and evaluation.

Identifying what learning has taken place

Group members usually learn a great deal by being involved in the discussion of someone's work. Therefore it is useful to make explicit what general learning has taken place from the specifics discussed, even if not all members bring something on every occasion.

Evaluation

All members evaluate the session at the end on a number of factors. These factors can be decided by the group, but may usefully include members' satisfaction with the process of selecting who works and for how long. Also all members can rate themselves on their level of participation, risk taken and their satisfaction with that. It can be helpful to use a scale from, say, 1 to 5. If this is done at the end of every session and a record is kept, it will over time give a clear indication of how the group is functioning. The result of this quick evaluation can be included in the 'what' section of the next session as it may influence how people decide to work. For example, someone may feel unhappy with their own level of defensiveness and lack of risk-taking and ask the group for help with this.

USEFUL TOOLS AND TECHNIQUES

Group supervision is different. Although the supervision can be carried out in a similar way to one-to-one supervision, I think it is a pity if this is always done. There are a variety of models, tools and techniques, which are easier or more effective if used with a group. Some groups like to have the kind of working agreement that allows for experimentation with a range of models and techniques. For example, they may decide that at regular intervals they devote a session to trying out something new. Such openness to different methods has the advantages of keeping the group lively and broadening everyone's experience. The tools and techniques introduced in this section are set out according to the 3-Step format, which makes them easy to implement.

THE DISCUSSION METHOD
Step 1: What is the issue?

1. The supervisee is chosen by whatever method the group feels comfortable with.
2. The supervisee explains the issue and what outcome she would like from the session.
3. Each group member is given the opportunity to ask a question for clarification or further information.

Step 2: How will it be worked with?

1. The group is facilitated to discuss the supervisee's issue.
2. The supervisee sits slightly outside the group and does not take part.
3. The discussion can either be for a reasonable length of time, say 30 minutes, or can be done in two or three sections.
4. After each discussion the supervisee is asked what she noticed, thought or felt. Were there any surprises?

Step 3: What Now?

1. The supervisee is asked how she sees the issue now. Has the desired outcome been achieved?

2. Group members evaluate the process and state what has been learnt.

THE INCIDENT METHOD
Step 1: What is the issue?

1. Each member is asked to bring a problematic incident to supervision.

2. Each person briefly describes the incident.

3. The facilitator asks each member to rank the incidents according to interest or usefulness for the supervision.

4. The facilitator helps the group to choose the incident to be worked on.

5. The person whose incident has been chosen (the supervisee) first describes it in more detail and then states what outcome they would like from its analysis.

Step 2: How will it be worked with?

1. Each group member writes one or more questions, preferably on a flip chart or large sheet of paper, as this will prevent duplication.

2. The facilitator helps the supervisee to answer and reflect on each question in turn.

3. The facilitator summarises the reflection or invites a group member to do so.

Step 3: What Now?

1. Each member is asked to state his or her view of the situation.

2. The supervisee is asked how they see things now and (if appropriate) what action they intend to take.

3. General discussion – approximately 10–15 minutes.

4. Each member evaluates the session and states what has been learnt.

CHOOSING A THEME

Step 1: What is the theme?

1. Each member states a 'theme' they would like discussed.
2. The facilitator or a group member makes notes on a flip chart or large sheet of paper.
3. The facilitator reads out each theme.
4. The group chooses one or more themes to work on.

Step 2: How will it be worked on?

1. Each member states their question related to the theme, which is noted on a flip chart.
2. The group is facilitated to work on one question at a time.
3. Each member is asked to engage with the question, using concrete examples from their own experience. This can take the form of several 'rounds'.

Step 3: What Now?

1. Each member states what has been learnt and what specific action they may take.
2. Each member evaluates the session.

CREATIVE FORCE FIELD ANALYSIS

This method is particularly suited to complicated work situations that feel frozen or stuck and where the way forward is unclear.

Step 1: What are the issues?

1. Each member is asked to draw or paint his or her situation (10–15 minutes). If people do not like drawing or painting they can try 'rapid writing' (see Chapter 4).
2. People split up into pairs and take turns to talk about their drawing (10 minutes).
3. The drawings are placed in a circle; each member very briefly explains their drawing (2–3 minutes each).
4. The facilitator helps the group to choose a situation to work on. (For some people the activity of drawing and talking about it can be sufficient to achieve a different view.)

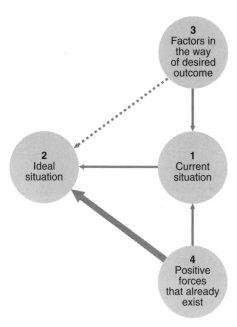

Figure 9.1   Force field analysis.

Step 2: How does force field analysis work?

1. The chosen drawing, representing the current situation, is placed in the centre of a large sheet of paper and a circle is drawn around it. The supervisee explains the situation briefly. Members suggest a short phrase or metaphor that (to the supervisee) describes the situation succinctly. The phrase or metaphor is written below the drawing. Three further circles are drawn and the numbers 2, 3 and 4 inserted (see Fig. 9.1).

2. The supervisee is asked how she would like the situation to be ideally. Sometimes the situation is so stuck that this is difficult for the supervisee to do. Group members can help the supervisee by, for example, asking the 'miracle question',[1] asking the supervisee to visualise her ideal situation or any other method that occurs. The outcome is written in circle 2.

---

[1]The 'miracle question' involves asking the supervisee to imagine that while she was asleep during the night a miracle has occurred and the situation has been resolved. What would be different? How would she know? What would she be feeling, thinking? What would she be doing differently?

3. Next, group members help the supervisee identify all the factors that get in the way of achieving her desired outcome. The answers to this are listed in circle 3.

4. Group members then help the supervisee identify positive forces that already exist, that would help their vision (circle 2) to happen, if only the restraining forces (circle 3) were not there. If it is difficult to identify positive forces, the supervisee may be asked to think of anything that does not make the situation worse.

Step 3: What Now?

1. Group members help the supervisee identify how each of the restraining forces could be reduced a little. This is written next to each force in a third colour.

2. Group members help the supervisee identify how each positive force could be enhanced a little. This is written next to each force in a fourth colour.

3. The group looks at the four circles and each member adds anything that comes to mind that may be useful. This may be written in a second colour.

4. The supervisee is helped to develop a concrete plan from points 1 and 2, which should include prioritising and time limits.

5. Each group member evaluates the session and states one thing that they have learnt.

A force field analysis can be adapted for more personal work issues, in which case the restraining forces may be renamed 'weaknesses or qualities' which their supervisee wants to see less of. Positive forces could be renamed strengths or qualities that the supervisee would like to see more of.

REFLECTION THROUGH RELAXATION
Step 1: What is the issue?

1. The supervisee describes a difficult situation and outlines what he would like to gain from the session.

Step 2: How will the issue be reflected on?

The facilitator asks for a 10-minute silence, during which each group member, including the supervisee, ponders on the issue. It is helpful if the facilitator leads the exercise as follows:

Sit in a comfortable position with both feet on the floor and close your eyes. Breathe gently and evenly ... Let yourself become aware of your body and not the position of every part ... If you come across any tension just say to that part 'release and relax ...' Now imagine yourself in the situation just described. Do not try to find a solution, but let yourself simply be there. Let any thoughts that appear simply come and go, without dwelling on them. If you find yourself drifting off, bring yourself back to the problem situation.

After 10 minutes bring the group back by saying:

Begin to breathe a little deeper now. In a few moments I am going to count to three and on the count of three you may open your eyes and have a bit of a stretch. One ... two ... three.

The relaxation is followed by people sharing their thoughts and feelings.

Step 3: What Now?

1. The supervisee is asked how he thinks and feels about the situation now and what he might do differently.

2. All group members are asked to briefly evaluate the session and to identify their own points of learning.

MASK-MAKING

It is good if sufficient time can be given to this method – at least 1½–2 hours. Mask-making materials need to be available: stiff paper or card, paints, glue, glitter, felt tips, scissors, rubber bands or ribbon for tying the masks on.

Step 1: What is the issue?

The facilitator first relaxes the group by saying the following:

Sit in a comfortable position with both feet on the floor and close your eyes. Breathe gently and evenly ... Let yourself become aware of your body and not the position of every part ... If you come across any tension just say to that part 'release and relax ...'

Now think of a client you are currently working with. See her very clearly, see the environment in which you usually see her, where are you placed, where does she sit? What are you both wearing? How does she look to you? What is the face she presents? ... Now imagine that you can look below the surface. What is your fantasy of the face you cannot see, the face that your client may not even know about herself? In a few moments I will invite you to create two masks, one for each face of the client – the face you see and the face that is hidden. Try not to speak too much while you are doing this ... you have plenty of time to do this ... In a few moments I am going to count to three; on the count of three you may open your eyes and, without speaking, take whatever materials you need and make your masks.

People make their masks.

Step 2: How will the masks be used to reflect?

How this is done will depend on the size of the group, but what tends to work quite well is the following format.

1. People split up in groups of three, and are given a letter – A, B or C.

2. A role-plays her own client and dons the masks that represents the 'seen' face.

3. B is her counsellor and they have a 5-minute session, while C observes.

4. Supervision session: C supervises B while A listens.

5. A role-plays her client wearing the 'unseen' mask and is counselled by B.

6. C supervises B while A listens.

Step 3: What Now?

1. A is debriefed and shares her experience of how being the client has deepened her understanding, and how she might proceed working with this client.

2. All three reflect on their experience of the exercise and state what has been learnt.

If there is time, Steps 2 and 3 can be repeated with different people role-playing their clients.

VISUALISATION

This method is particularly useful for exploring what happened between a worker and a client.

Step 1: What is the issue?

1. The supervisee is chosen by whatever method has been decided.

2. Next the supervisee explains the issue briefly and what outcome she would like from the session.

Step 2: How will the issue be reflected on?

1. The facilitator says to the supervisee, 'Visualise yourself as the relationship between you and your client and speak from that'. So you start with 'I am the relationship between ...' etc. Some people find it helpful to close their eyes for this, but it is not essential.

2. Group members can ask questions such as 'Tell me ... relationship', 'How do you feel about ...?' etc.

Step 3: What Now?

1. When questions dry up the supervisee is asked, as herself, what the experience was like for her. How does she see things now? What might she do differently?

2. It may be necessary to debrief the supervisee by asking her to state that she is not the relationship, and to say her name and perhaps her profession.

3. Each group member is asked to evaluate the session and to state what has been learnt.

This method may be adapted in several ways: the supervisee may visualise herself as the client, the client's problem, the difficult situation in the client's life, a difficult situation in the supervisee's work place, and so on.

SCULPTING

This method is useful for a complicated organisational situation or for getting a sense of relationship patterns in the life of a client.

Step 1: What is the issue?

1. The supervisee is chosen by whatever method the group has agreed.

2. The supervisee briefly describes the situation, the relationships within it and the people involved.

3. Group members ask any questions they need for clarification.

Step 2: How is the issue worked with?

1. The supervisee chooses people to play particular roles.

2. The facilitator helps the group to create a 'sculpt' which for the supervisee represents the situation accurately. (In a sculpt people do not move, but stand or sit in a way that fits the character they occupy. Also where they are in the sculpt in relation to each other should reflect those roles and relationships.)

3. Each person is asked to speak as his or her character. What are they thinking, feeling?

4. What is it like to be occupying that place? What do they want?

5. Group members not taking a role state their reactions to the sculpt.

Step 3: What Now?

1. The supervisee gives his reactions to the sculpt? How does he see things now?

2. Can he see a way forward? What actions might he take?

3. People in the sculpt give their opinion of the supervisee's proposed actions.

4. This may be enough, or it may lead to the supervisee modifying his proposed actions.

5. The sculpt is disbanded and each person is debriefed by stating 'I am not ..., I am ... (their own name)'.

6. Each member evaluates the session and states what has been learnt.

ROLE-PLAY

Like sculpting, this method is suited to the exploration of situations involving complicated relationships. Special sessions can be set aside for this method so that group members can come prepared with suitable situations. Alternatively, the group may like to use it as and when it seems suitable to what the supervisee brings.

Step 1: What is the issue?

1. The supervisee is chosen by whatever method has been decided.

2. The supervisee explains the situation and what outcome she would like from the session.

3. Each group is given the opportunity to ask a question for clarification or further information.

Step 2: How will the reflection and role-play be conducted?

1. The supervisee chooses people to play the various roles and briefs each person on their role until they are clear. It may be necessary for the supervisee to do brief demonstrations re body posture, way of speaking, etc.

2. If the supervisee is involved in the situation she first plays herself.

3. Next, another member plays the supervisee with the supervisee watching.

4. The supervisee may play several other roles if this is likely to be useful.

5. After every brief role-play each participant says what he or she is thinking and feeling.

Step 3: What Now?

1. The facilitator and other group members give feedback on what they have noticed.

2. The supervisee says how she feels now, has a shift occurred? Are there any actions she would like to take? Does she want to do another brief role-play?

3. Role-playing group members are debriefed by stating 'I am not ... I am ... (their name).'

4. All group members evaluate the session and state what has been learnt.

REFLECTION BY INTERVIEW
Step 1: What is the issue?

This method is particularly useful for anyone who works with clients one-to-one and would like to reflect on how the work is going.

1. The supervisee gives a brief synopsis of the history with the client and what outcome they would like from the session.

Step 2: How will the reflection be conducted?

1. The supervisee role-plays his client and one or more group members interview him. The questions they ask may include:
—How is the counselling going?
—What are you getting from it?
—What would you like that you are not getting?
—What do you think of your counsellor?
—What do you imagine he thinks about you?
—How would you describe your relationship?
—What would you really like to say to him but feel you can't?
—Any other questions that members feel may be useful.
2. Other group members watch and observe their own feelings and reactions.
3. After the interview people share their thoughts and feelings.

Step 3: What Now?

1. The supervisee is debriefed: 'I am not ... but I am ...'
2. The supervisee shares how he sees things now. Has the desired outcome been achieved?
3. What action would he now like to take?
4. Group members evaluate the process and state what has been learnt.

REFLECTING ON UNCONSCIOUS DYNAMICS

In Chapter 6 I discussed how the psychodynamic approach to supervision is concerned with the identification and illumination of unconscious processes such as transferences, projections and parallels. These processes may be experienced in the therapeutic space between practitioner and client as well as in the supervision space, between supervisor and supervisee. When we are in the grip of a transference or a projection we may not be aware of it; that is the nature of the beast. On the other hand, these processes can seem much more obvious when they happen to someone else. This is where group supervision is useful, as we can learn a great deal from the observation of unconscious processes in other people.

TASK AND MAINTENANCE

A supervision group needs to pay attention, both to its task and to its maintenance. The task involves the actual supervision itself and should receive most of the group's attention. Maintenance should not be ignored, however, as it gives the group the opportunity to reflect on its own process. It should, therefore, always form a part of Step 3 of the supervision.

Task

When reflecting on unconscious dynamics it is good to do this without attaching 'rights' or 'wrongs', but instead maintaining a spirit of respectful enquiry. Also, it is good not to get attached to our ideas or intuitions, but to treat them as hypotheses – to be tested out (if appropriate) through the continued work between practitioner and client. The supervision may be seen as a space where those ideas and hunches may be played with, thrown around like a ball, caught, dropped, thrown in the air again, discarded for another one, and so on. What I am saying is that it is good to hold our hypotheses lightly, so that at all times we remain open to other ideas.

It is an interesting phenomenon that different group members often pick up different aspects, both of the client's internal world and of the worker–client relationship. If a group works well, the outcome of a session may involve a 'consensus about networks of connections in the patient's material,' giving it a 'deeper meaning and dimension' (Kalsched in Kugler 1995:111).

The task of supervision can be accomplished in a number of different ways, depending on such factors as the maturity of the group, the leadership style of the facilitator, or the work context of the group members. Unless participants are already used to focusing on their own responses while listening to a supervisee's account of their work, it may be useful to start off with a fairly authoritarian style.

I attended a supervision workshop led by Robin Shohet, where the following formula was used: The facilitator starts working with the supervisee, while the other group members stay silent and are asked to focus only on their own thoughts, emotions or physical responses or experiences. From time to time the facilitator stops and asks each group member in turn to say only what he or she experienced as they listened to the supervisee. This can be difficult at times, as people often want to say more or want to start analysing what they think is going on. So it is important that the facilitator really holds on to their authority. When all have spoken the facilitator summarises what was said and asks the supervisee to continue, and to say, if they want, their responses to what people said. After a set amount of time, ideally 5 or 10 minutes before the supervisee's allocated time is up, there can be a more general sharing and feedback.

Since attending that workshop with Robin Shohet, I have taught and practised this way of working with many different kinds of groups. Invariably I am struck by how accurately different group members seem to experience different aspects of the psychodynamics of the client, the supervisee or the relationship between the two. Even sheepish comments such as 'Sorry, I lost concentration, I was miles away,' or 'I was distracted by the noise of people outside' are often found to be relevant.

Kalsched warns against (premature) searching for too much clarity or abstraction in group supervision (Kalsched in Kugler 1995:113). Similarly, Brookes advocates a spirit of 'subjectivity and open-endedness rather than objectivity' (Brookes in Kugler 1995:121). This is because our internal worlds as well as our interactions are much more complex than meets the eye. In supervision (and maybe also in our work with clients) we try and make the unconscious conscious, or, to use a metaphor, to bring what is dark into the light. However, we should not forget that the part of the iceberg that is underneath the water is larger and goes deeper than we are ever able to comprehend. Realising this may help us to refrain from thinking that now we understand everything that there is to know about someone or about a relationship. Hopefully it will keep us humble and aware that ultimately there will always be much that remains a mystery about each and every one of us.

Maintenance

We all know that groups are breeding grounds for unconscious processes, including projections, splitting, acting out, to say nothing of dysfunctional family dynamics such as sibling rivalry, envy, scapegoating, co-dependency, etc. (Kalsched in Kugler 1995:111)

As is clear from the above quote, we all have a dark side and a supervision group is no exception. Although the primary function of the group is the task of providing supervision for its members, a good facilitator will also build in space for 'maintenance', where the dark side can be illuminated and explored. In Step 1 the 'what' of the session needs to be agreed. What is going to be the focus, task or maintenance? If a group is not working well, it would seem a good idea to spend a session reflecting on what might be going on. However, this will be uncomfortable and may meet with resistance or antagonism from some if not all members. The supervisor needs to be skilled to deal with this situation. I believe that an 'up-front' approach is often the best policy. For example, a supervisor might say, 'I think it would be a good idea for us to look at how we are functioning as it is my impression that we are not working well. I guess that some of the reluctance may be about fearing what may be exposed. There are two things I should like to say about that. First, what we fear is often far worse than what actually happens. Second, we are not working well, and I am therefore not sure how useful a "task"- oriented session would be – it could even be damaging.' This is likely to lead to more discussion and hopefully agreement. Of course, it is possible that, for whatever reason, the group does not want to look at itself on that occasion, perhaps because one or two participants feel that they really need supervision that day. In that case it would be good to agree a 'maintenance' session for a specific date. This means that the problem is not allowed to go underground, where it would continue to fester and disrupt the working of the group. It gives group members the opportunity to think about the situation and reflect on what they think is happening in the meantime. It also means that the facilitator has retained her authority, which is important if the group is going to continue.

The 'owning' of personal experience

A maintenance session needs to be well facilitated and benefits from an honest and straightforward approach. This means that each person speaks from their own experience only, using 'I' statements, such as: 'I am aware of feeling a bit frustrated when you said ...,' or 'I felt a sense of irritation when you said ...,' or 'I am finding it difficult to engage with this ... But I am not sure why that is.' When people 'own their own experience' like this it sounds quite different from saying 'You make me feel frustrated,' or 'You are so irritating.' Other useful rules to observe include:

- Only one person speaks at any one time.
- All take the time to listen to each other.
- All endeavour to observe what is going on for themselves.

 EXAMPLE OF A BRIEF DIALOGUE

John: Just now, I thought that Fred did not really answer Sally's question. I felt annoyed at that and I would like to know how you felt Sally?

Sally: No, I don't feel like that. I did think Fred answered the question I asked.

Tina: I feel uncomfortable as if I am missing something. I have a feeling that something is happening that I cannot put my finger on and I don't know what it is. I would like to know whether anyone else feels like that?

John: I am wondering whether I misunderstood Sally's question. I thought you asked ...

Tina: I feel annoyed now. I just asked a question and it is being ignored.

John: Sorry Tina, I felt excited just now as if I'm on to something. Actually, I am also wondering whether you actually misunderstood Sally's question.

Tina: I feel frustrated, as we don't seem to be getting to the point. I want to ask you Sally – could you ask the question again and say what you meant by it?

Sally: Sure, I asked ... by which I meant ... Is that clearer now?

John: Yes, thanks, I had misunderstood.

Facilitator: I am aware that this kind of thing has happened
before – with Tina and John not understanding what
Sally is saying. I also notice John, that you cut across
Tina twice ... and so on.

As this example hopefully demonstrates everyone speaks in a non-reactive way and thinks before they speak. In addition, each person is committed to honesty and to working with the 'here and now', rather than what happened in the group's past.

Other methods

Some of the methods outlined in the previous section of this chapter may also be used to work on the maintenance of the group. For example, all group members could be given the opportunity to create a group 'sculpt' according to how they see the group. Each person then says how he or she feels in that position. Once all members have created their sculpt everyone should be much clearer on how different members see things, which should be helpful in finding a solution.

Alternatively, all create a painting or drawing of how they see themselves in relation to the group. Again, once each member has shared their perception, the route is paved towards developing a way forward.

Of course, there does not need to be a crisis for these kinds of methods to be useful. A well-functioning group should have maintenance built in as part of its normal process. As demonstrated earlier in this chapter, I like to build in a review of the process of supervision into Step 3 of every session. In any case, it is good practice for regular review to be built into the group's working agreement, as part of a more general commitment to evaluation of the supervision's effectiveness.

CONCLUSION

In this chapter I discussed how the 3-Step method may be used both in the setting up and the running of a supervision group. Groups lend themselves well to the use of creative methods, so in the next section I included a range of different tools and techniques. Lastly, I discussed the importance of bringing unconscious dynamics into awareness, both for the task and for the maintenance of the supervision group.

Questions for further reflection

- What experiences have you had of group supervision?
- Do you now see these experiences in a different light?
- If so, what in particular has made a difference?
- If you have not so far participated in a supervision group, what are your thoughts and feelings about it?
- Would you like to try group supervision? If so, what is it that you would like to get out of it?

10

Some thoughts on management, leadership and supervision in organisations

*Many supervisees need help with organisational dynamics
and relations with their professional team.*
(Bramley 1996:22)

*Self-growth is tender. It's holy ground. There is no
greater investment.* (Covey 1992:62)

In this chapter I first share some of my thoughts about the general usefulness of supervision as well as its relationship to management and leadership. I then discuss some ideas for the provision of a transformational style of leadership. Lastly, I outline how the 3-Step method can be used to implement supervision within an organisation.

CLINICAL SUPERVISION AS PART OF CONTINUOUS PERSONAL AND PROFESSIONAL DEVELOPMENT

*An educational process always extends over a substantial
period of time – typically a lifetime.*
(Speicher in Kugler 1995:193)

Within the helping professions the concept of continuous professional (as well as personal) development is increasingly recognised as essential to the maintenance and enhancement of practice. Some professions, such as nursing or counselling, will renew people's registration or accreditation only if they have fulfilled a requisite amount of developmental activities. Implicit in this requirement is the idea that knowledge is not static and that we can never rest on our laurels. Ideally, it is not just institutional requirements that prompt people to attend workshops, study days, conferences or courses. In order to have job satisfaction most of us need to feel that we do our work well and that we are effective. And, in order to be effective we need to continue learning. It is a funny thing, but it is not the case that once we stop learning we stay at the same level. We don't, we stagnate and stagnation will inevitably lead to deterioration.

Some years ago I looked at the names given to horses taking part in the Grand National. The name of one horse particularly struck me. It was 'Rust Never Sleeps'. The horse did not win the race and I lost my (very small) bet. However, the name has really stuck with me as a useful reminder that if we do not keep up with current professional knowledge and developments we get rusty. Those of us who engage in DIY, car maintenance or gardening know that it is important to look after our tools and prevent them from getting rusty, as rusty tools make the job more difficult if not impossible. It is therefore a good habit to clean our tools after use and to oil them regularly. In the helping professions we, ourselves, are the tools. It is how we are and how we do what we do that makes the difference. Clinical supervision is a good way, metaphorically speaking, to prevent us from getting rusty.

CLINICAL SUPERVISION AS PART OF A PROCESS OF TRANSFORMATION

For any organisation, but particularly for those concerned with helping people, the effectiveness of its workforce, which is often its main asset, is of paramount importance. Clinical supervision can be part of the way in which this asset is maintained and cared for. Effectiveness, whether at the personal or the organisational level, is a matter of balancing short-term goals with long-term goals and objectives. One of the long-term objectives of a hospital, for example, may be to have a workforce that is happy and stable, with a low turnover and sickness rate. In the short term, however, staff shortages and perennial financial concerns may cause the management to over-focus on short-term solutions, shelving the long-term goals to be dealt with when times are better. This is an example of an effectiveness imbalance (Covey 1992:59). Shelving or sacrificing long-term objectives for more immediate concerns may not only create more problems than it solves, it may also make the realisation of the long-term goal more difficult.

For example, at times of personnel shortages hospitals focus on solving the immediate problem by staffing their clinical areas with agency staff, often at great expense. This may then mean that there is no money available for the implementation of schemes that might help attract and retain staff. Clinical supervision can be part of such a scheme if it is implemented in a way that makes people feel supported and cared for. For clinical supervision to be perceived in such a positive manner, the long-term objective must be kept in mind. This implies adequate investment and ongoing resourcing and setting up a sound infrastructure in terms of supervision time built into the working week, suitable spaces and adequate training and preparation for supervision.

THE IMPORTANCE OF ADEQUATE INVESTMENT

Within healthcare, many hospital trusts have set a finite sum of money aside for the implementation of clinical supervision, some-times as a 'one-off' initiative. A nurse or occupational therapist, for example, may be appointed for a 6- or 12-month period and charged with the task of implementing clinical supervision throughout the trust. I have noticed that such posts are often not at a very high man-agerial level, which could mean that the post holder might be per-ceived as lacking the necessary authority. Also, it is debatable to what extent one person can successfully carry out such a mammoth task in limited time. In my view, unless the investment in the imple-mentation of clinical supervision is adequate and ongoing, it is unlikely to produce the desired result. In the long run an inadequate investment in clinical supervision is false economy. It may also have a negative effect on the workforce, who may doubt the sincerity of its management and see them as only paying lip service to the idea of clinical supervision and continuous professional development. There can be a mismatch between what is espoused in an organisa-tion's official policy on supervision and its 'low-profile symbols', how it is actually implemented and the actual importance placed upon it (Hawkins & Shohet 2000:168).

It is really helpful if an organisation can foster an atmosphere of containment and challenge. In such an organisation people are more likely to respond to the challenge of clinical supervision with enthusiasm, as they feel contained by the organisation providing sufficient resources and training. Also, an organisation which encourages people to have a go at clinical supervision and which allows mistakes to be made, is more likely to have a successful scheme going before long. This is because allowing mistakes and valuing them as a useful source of learning, frees people up to try out various models of implementation and practice, in order to discover what works best for them.

THE RELATIONSHIP BETWEEN MANAGEMENT, SUPERVISION AND LEADERSHIP

The very basis of real leadership is selflessness. (Hawley 1993)

Styles of management and leadership are believed to be associated, not only with people's feelings of job satisfaction and wellbeing, but also with the quality of service they provide to their clients (Carlowe 1998, Thomas 1998, Williams et al 1998). Lack of management support can lead to high rates of sickness and absenteeism, as well as problems in recruitment and retention (Williams et al 1998).

OPTIONS FOR IMPLEMENTATION

I believe that clinical supervision can be part of a transformational style of management and leadership. As far as its implementation is concerned, there appear to be three main options:

1. All supervision is managerial.
2. Managers provide managerial supervision, clinical supervisors provide clinical supervision.
3. All supervision is non-managerial.

I personally believe that it is a good idea for people to have clinical supervision from an outsider in addition to supervision from their manager. Although I have written elsewhere about the undesirability of all supervision being provided by managers (van Ooijen 2000:26–31), I have shifted my position slightly in the realisation that the effectiveness of the supervision is contingent upon the actual quality of the working relationship between the supervisor and the supervisee. From my discussions with many people throughout the country, I know that, if that relationship is good and both parties value, respect and trust each other, managerial supervision can work very well. But where that relationship is not as good as it might be, the inherent power imbalance can lead to many problems. For example, it may prevent supervisees from being honest and they hide the very aspects of their work they should be bringing to supervision because they want to create a good impression.

For this reason some organisations prefer to create a supervision system that is not managerial. In this case it may be advisable to develop very clear working agreements or contracts so that everyone is clear who is responsible for what. Some organisations may like a regular report from the supervisor, which would need to be clearly and carefully negotiated with the supervisees. If this is not done it could defeat the object of the non-managerial nature of the supervision completely, as people may feel unsafe and not trust that the information will be treated confidentially. In order to feel safe, supervisees are likely to want to know what is the purpose of the report, what information is asked for, who will read it, etc. I have come across people who claimed that their supervisor had to write a report of all supervision sessions, which was then sent to various levels in the hierarchy without any guarantee of confidentiality. It is hard to see how this type of supervision could possibly be effective, as the supervisees were obviously very selective in what they talked about. However, where all parties concerned are in agreement, the report can actually form part of the evaluation of the effectiveness of supervision at organisational level. As discussed in Chapter 7, supervisees are usually happy to write the report together with their supervisor and to focus on how useful they feel the supervision is and what concrete outcomes have been achieved.

THE IMPORTANCE OF THE MANAGERIAL ROLE

It seems to me that, even if all clinical supervision is provided within a non-managerial context, there still needs to be leadership, indeed supervision, provided by the manager. After all, managers do need to have a sense of their staff: who they are as people and professionals, the standard of their work, how they are developing and any aspirations and ideas or problems that they may have. It can therefore be useful to have the clinical supervision provided by someone other than the manager, leaving the manager free to provide the more managerial supervision and to keep a handle on the quality of the work that is provided by their staff. However, as discussed in Chapter 2, the ground rules of the working agreement must be set in tablets of stone. This means that, if it has been agreed to meet on the first Tuesday afternoon of every month, then it is vital that both parties stick to this arrangement. Cancelling supervision, for whatever reason, may give the staff member the message that they are not important and are only fitted in when the manager has nothing better to do. Having regular, protected time with staff can provide managers with a system for keeping in touch with them. Particularly if people are also having clinical supervision from someone outside the management structure, supervision sessions with their manager can have a different emphasis. For example, the clinical supervision sessions may be used to focus on particular work situations, such as relationships with clients or the handling of a particular problem. Managerial supervision, on the other hand, could lean more towards developing staff as professionals. In other words, incorporate some elements of professional coaching (Parsloe 1999).

Whichever style of implementation is chosen, the role of the manager remains crucial to the well-being of the staff. For example, it is possible to think of some people feeling very supported by their (non-managerial) supervisor; they feel they are also learning a great deal and feel that their practice is improving greatly. Because of the way they are developing both personally and professionally, they start to question the way certain things are done in the organisation and are coming up with ideas for improvement. At this point the manager plays an important role.

UNHELPFUL MANAGERIAL ATTITUDES

Ideally, managers will be supportive of their staff's development and see this as synonymous with best practice and the improvement of the service to the clients. If managers are truly committed to clinical supervision and to the development of their staff, supervision and management will work hand in hand for the benefit of all concerned: the clients, the organisation and the supervisee. If this is not the case, however, supervision may be seen as a nuisance or a threat, or interfering with 'the work'. If this is the case, subtle obstacles may be placed in the way of supervision. For example, people may be given urgent work to do at the time when they have a supervision appointment, or they may be told that it is a luxury that the department cannot afford at the moment.

Also, particularly in some helping professions, there can be a tendency to try to cut down those who stand out from the rest. Sometimes managers feel so overwhelmed by the demands of their job that they become demotivated and have no interest in the ideas their staff may come up with, or they may even see their staff's development as a direct threat to themselves.

BOUNDARY PROBLEMS

Another problem that can occur when the clinical supervisor is also the supervisee's manager is a lack of boundaries. For example, it would clearly be undesirable to accost a supervisee on the stairs or in the corridor in order to have a quick update on Mr so-and-so. This breaks an ethical boundary (Bramley 1996:155). Not only is there a danger of confidential information being overheard, but also it is not fair to expect someone to give an instant opinion without preparation. It certainly would not be in the client's best interest. Lastly, such 'breaks' in the frame of supervision make it very unsafe, as it is no longer kept within the agreed boundaries. If I had a supervisor/manager who expected me to engage in quick consultations outside the supervision sessions I would think, 'What else can she not keep confidential?' Although supervision is about our work, inevitably our supervisor will get to know a great deal about us in that role. Therefore the thought that a manager/supervisor could not be trusted would be very damaging.

UNHELPFUL ORGANISATIONAL DYNAMICS

In the chapters on the 'how' of supervision I have written about the importance of paying attention to the 'unconscious' or the 'non-rational' in people's individual experience. An organisation has an unconscious element too, which is expressed within its culture and organisational dynamics (Hawkins & Shohet 2000:169). For supervision to work well within an organisation its culture needs to be favourable. If the culture is unhealthy, it is likely that supervision will be affected accordingly. Either it will be allowed simply to disappear, or it will be used in a way that is unlikely to achieve best practice.

Hawkins and Shohet have identified five unhelpful cultural dynamics and the effect they have on how supervision is implemented and experienced:

- Hunt the personal pathology.
- Strive for bureaucratic efficiency.
- Watch your back.
- Driven by crisis.
- The addictive organisation.

(Hawkins & Shohet 2000:170–176)

I have renamed these dynamics as follows:

- Find the scapegoat.
- The checklist approach.
- Trust no-one.
- Crisis gets you attention.
- Addicted? Moi?

Find the scapegoat When problems occur in an organisation with this dynamic they tend to be seen as caused by a particular person, who then becomes the scapegoat. 'If only "so-and-so" would leave, everything would be fine' is the general attitude. Supervision may be seen as only relevant in case of problems and unnecessary when 'things are fine'.

The checklist approach Here the focus is on 'checking that all the tasks have been done', which may leave little or no time for reflection or support. The supervisor may use an actual checklist that they work through during the session.

Trust no-one Here the climate may be very competitive or politicised with many factions and subgroups. Supervisees tend to feel that it is not safe to admit to problems or worries and may cover up anything that they are not sure about.

Crisis gets you attention In many of the helping professions the workload is so high and people so stressed that the only way in which its users may get attention is by producing a crisis. Alternatively, staff may only be given attention by their manager in case of a crisis. Supervision is unlikely to be a priority in this culture and sessions will get cancelled whenever there is something else going on that is regarded as more important (which will be very often).

Addicted? Moi?   Hawkins and Shohet identify four kinds of addictive organisation:

- Someone in a key position is an addict.
- Many of its staff replicate addictive or co-dependent patterns.
- The organisation itself is the source of addiction – e.g. workaholism is a requirement.
- The organisation itself demonstrates the characteristic of an addictive personality – rationalising rather than facing difficulties.

In supervision it may be difficult to get people to be honest; however, 'denial and dishonesty' must be interrupted for it to be effective (Hawkins & Shohet 2000:174–175).

COMBINED CULTURAL DYNAMICS

Sometimes several dynamics can operate at once, such as 'Addicted? Moi?' and 'Find the scapegoat'. I once encountered a team where no-one appeared to talk to each other much – the message was that they were all far too busy for that. If a newcomer felt that they needed to ask people questions about how things were done, indeed, about what they should actually be doing, they would quickly get the message that they were expected to 'just get on with it'. Coffee, tea or lunch breaks did not seem to happen either and everyone stayed on for much longer than they were paid for. However, even though people did not appear to talk much in public, there was also a scapegoating culture that went on behind the scenes. At regular intervals one person would be identified as a 'problem' and would be eased out by a number of different methods: making life difficult for them, giving them a very high workload, freezing them out, making official complaints, etc. Eventually this person would leave, after which things seemed to settle down for a while. Sooner or later though, someone else – not necessarily the person who had replaced the one who had left – would become a scapegoat, and the whole cycle started again.

Clearly this was a very sick team, and yet there was a system of team supervision in operation. However, it was not given importance and only happened when everyone could spare the time, which was not often. Also, sessions tended to be cancelled at the last minute when the manager needed to go to a high-level meeting, which meant that people almost expected not to have to turn up. The supervision sessions that did take place tended to be characterised by people either not really saying what was on their mind, or 'speaking in riddles', making vague accusations, which they then refused to clarify. Generally team members felt that they were far too busy to engage in something so unimportant as supervision and that anyway, 'so-and-so' was the real problem behind everything and should be got rid of – what was supervision supposed to achieve?

TRANSFORMING A TEAM

Managers can do much to counteract dysfunctional dynamics in their team, although this task can be very difficult if the whole organisation is dysfunctional, as what goes wrong within a team can often be a reflection of what is wrong within the organisation as a whole. In such cases it may be advisable to seek supervision from someone outside the organisation, who is experienced in the field of dysfunctional dynamics. In any case, change will only be effective if, firstly, staff feel that what they are already doing well is appreciated and, secondly, if they can 'own' their problems rather than denying their existence or trying to pass them on to others (Hawkins & Shohet 2000:183).

Managers who are committed to their team's development and who want to transform its dynamics need to focus on the individuals within their team (as well as on the team as a whole) in order to help them to:

- Be motivated
- Feel empowered
- Feel confident
- Take responsibility
- Make decisions
- Solve problems.

 THINKING POINT

If you are a manager, to what extent would you say you already do this? What is your perception of the individuals within your team? How can you empower people to feel motivated, confident and responsible? If you are not a manager, to what extent do you feel that your manager is helping you to feel motivated, confident and responsible?

Motivation

Whether you are working as a manager, team member or supervisor, the ability to motivate is an important skill to develop. This is because in a supportive environment motivated people will flourish and develop the confidence to take whatever responsibility they are ready for. When asked what they want from their working life, many helping professionals would probably answer 'job satisfaction'. Therefore, facilitating an environment that is likely to lead to job satisfaction is in itself motivating. However, before we can motivate others, we need to start with ourselves.

 THINKING POINT

Take some time to ask yourself the following questions:

- What motivates me?
- How can I motivate myself to keep developing my practice?
- What do I need to do that I am not doing now?
- What conditions do I need to ensure for myself?
- How good am I at gaining people's cooperation?
- How do others view my skills in obtaining people's cooperation?

It is good to have a clear idea of what makes us tick. It can also be helpful to find out what makes other people tick, such as colleagues and friends. You may like to ask them the same questions. I am often struck by how different people are. Often, when things go wrong it is due to people having made the assumption that others will be motivated by the same things as themselves.

TEAM-BUILDING

This section focuses on managers in charge of a team, or supervisors who are asked to supervise a team, or indeed any group.

As a team or group supervisor, a manager or a member of a team you may also find it useful to ask yourself, your supervisees, your staff, or your colleagues the following questions:

- What do you like most about your job?
- What do you find the most challenging?
- What do you do to keep up-to-date with your skills and knowledge?

- What impresses you most about the people you work with?
- What personal qualities do you have that have helped you in your career so far?

Getting people to trust each other so that they feel free to discuss their answers can be a very useful team- or group-building exercise. It will help people to get to know and understand each other better, which is an important step towards getting a team to cooperate.

Some useful guidelines

If you want a team to work well, perhaps to discuss an important issue or to solve a problem there are a number of useful guidelines to bear in mind.

- First ask yourself 'What is my view?' and 'What are my aims?' It is important for you to be clear on this, as without clarity any team discussion is likely to deteriorate into confusion, which can then lead to people feeling demotivated.
- Ask each team member to state his or her answers to the questions you just asked yourself. This helps focus the responsibility on everyone within the team, thus helping them to feel involved and motivated.
- Respect other people's rights to have different points of view to your own.
- Work with the team to establish, first, areas where cooperation is good and second, areas where cooperation needs to be improved.
- Facilitate the team to come up with a solution.
- Give praise where it is due.
- Admit personal errors of judgement (but without dwelling on them).
- Prevent differences of opinion from disintegrating into argument by helping people to focus on the issue or problem rather than on personalities.
- Recognise, however, that a good team is able to handle disagreements and conflicts by bringing them out in the open, rather than letting them fester below the surface.
- If you have been engaged in solving a problem that necessitates some action, be sure that you know how you can tell when it has been solved.

- Facilitate a team agreement on observable indicators, as well as a date by which to review them.

In Chapter 9 I discuss in more detail how supervisors can work efficiently and creatively with groups or teams.

DIFFERENT STYLES OF SUPERVISION OR MANAGEMENT

Good supervisors and managers are able to adapt their skills to the needs of the individuals. As a general rule this will lie on a continuum from mentorship for people who lack experience, via supportive, to empowering for those who are very experienced. Figure 10.1 sets out the differences between the various styles. As you can see, a transformational leader is never directive, but aims to help all team members to feel empowered and reach their own full potential. It is now realised that a directive style is undesirable, even for trainees, as it fosters dependency and lack of motivation. The way to facilitate student practitioners as well as other workers to become motivated, independent practitioners is through mentorship, support and empowerment.

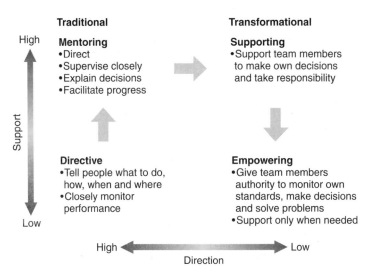

Figure 10.1 The different styles of supervision or management.

THINKING POINT

If you are managing or supervising a group or team, think of its members. Which style of leadership do you feel they need at the moment? Which style of leadership do you in turn require from those who support you?

Transformational leaders and supervisors carry their role lightly. This is because they believe in people's potential and are always looking to help people develop to their full capability. According to Hawley, leadership is about giving. This is how it differs from management, which he sees as seeking to 'get' things from people (Hawley 1993). So a transformational leader is a generous leader who will continuously aim to help people move along the cycle towards empowerment and independence.

Transformational leaders are wise leaders who, by keeping their self-interest in check, actually become far more effective than if they simply followed their own pursuits (Heider 1992). Similarly, empowered people are not threatened by the success of others. They work well together, secure in the knowledge that each person has their own sphere of authority, responsibility and expertise, but that support from the leader is available when required.

USING THE 3-STEP METHOD TO IMPLEMENT SUPERVISION

IMPLEMENTING SUPERVISION WITHIN A UNIT OR TEAM

Increasingly, senior people within the helping professions, such as nursing, the professions allied to medicine and many voluntary agencies, may not have experienced clinical supervision before but are becoming attracted to the idea of supervision as a useful vehicle for supporting, monitoring and developing their staff. It is not unusual for a manager to be told to 'implement' supervision within his or her team, but without much guidance as to how to go about it. In such cases the 3-Step method offers a simple framework to follow.

Box 10.1   The three steps to implementing supervision within a unit or team

---

Step 1: the 'what' of implementation

- What do I want to know about my staff so I can support them, facilitate their development and monitor their practice?

Step 2: the 'how' of implementation

- How am I going to find out?

Step 3: the 'what now' of implementation

- What am I going to do Now I have found out?

The three steps are outlined in Box 10.1 and are discussed in more detail in the following section.

Step 1: What do I want to know?

 THINKING POINT

Well, over to you. What is it that you feel you need to know about the people who report to you? If you are not a manager what do you think your manager would need to know in order to support, monitor and facilitate your development?

I find that the kinds of answers people come up with include the following:

- I need to have an idea of people's standard of work.
- I need to know how they feel about their work, not just how committed they are, but how well they feel they are doing.
- I need to know whether they feel that they are placed correctly or whether they might want to change their work.
- I need to know what they think about the unit/organisation.
- I need to know what they feel about me and my effectiveness as a manager; do they feel supported by me, or is there room for improvement?
- I need to know what they feel about the idea of clinical supervision.
- I need to know what they would like from supervision, what their own goals and objectives are, and what outcomes they would like.

- I need to know whether they feel good about having me as their main supervisor or would it be better to think of an alternative arrangement.
- I need to know what people's individual learning styles are.

And, perhaps most importantly:

- I need to know what my staff feel that I need to know.

You may well have thought of many additional areas that you would want to find out about. Really, it totally depends on you and the kind of area in which you and your staff work.

Step 2: How am I going to find out?

 THINKING POINT

How would you go about finding out what you need to know?

There are a number of ways in which a manager can find out the needed information and they all involve 'asking people'. However, there are different ways in which people can be asked. Also, organisations being what they are, people need to know – for their part – why you are asking them. So you need to be up-front about your own purposes, aims, goals and objectives in first of all wanting to implement clinical supervision, and, secondly, why you feel you need to have answers to these questions. It is not advisable to short-cut this step and to assume that you already know the answers. Take the example of learning styles. Sometimes people assume that everyone learns in the same way and that what works for them will therefore also work for everyone else. This assumption can be a recipe for disaster and lead to much frustration as not everyone learns in the same way. For example, I know that some people like to be given the responsibility to go and seek out information, whereas others learn more from watching someone else or from attending a lecture, or from being allowed to try things out again and again under supervision.

Matching learning styles

I personally experienced how frustrating it is when someone tries to teach you something in a way that does not fit your learning style. A friend offered to teach me how to play chess, as it was something I had always wanted to learn. She produced a chess-board and two pieces, one of which may have been the King, and proceeded to tell me all about the relationship between them and what moves were possible. She wanted me to practise this over and over until I had understood this thoroughly before adding more pieces. It did not work. Basically I am a 'top-down' person, who needs to know the broad sweep first, before I engage with the detail. Starting with the detail is impossible for me, as without relating it to the overall game it just does not make sense. My friend, on the other hand, has a 'bottom-up' learning style and thought that I was just being thick. For her, knowing the details first was the only way to learn.

Both learning styles are valid and both will work equally well, provided the learner and the style are matched. As I discovered, what does not work is to force people to use an approach that does not come naturally to them. Either it will not work at all, or it will be a very laborious process and take much longer than is necessary. In my case, one day while my children were choosing some books from the library, I found a book that aimed to teach children all about chess. It explained how the game had been developed and why the various pieces related to each other as they did. I was really pleased to find such a simple top-down approach that helped me to get a sense of what it was all about. Now I could begin to learn. I never became very good, in fact one of my sons picked it up much faster than I did – but that is a different story.

The moral of the story is that it makes good sense to match learning styles to the learner, as not to do so is neither efficient nor likely to be very effective.

Step 3: What am I going to do Now I have found out?

The implementation of supervision always needs careful preparation, whether at the level of individuals, an organisation or a professional team. As discussed earlier in the book, a great deal of preparatory work needs to be done before we can even begin supervision. Any job worth doing tends to need adequate preparation, and the implementation of clinical supervision is no different.

Box 10.2 Three steps to implementing clinical supervision in an organisation

Step 1: the 'what' of implementation
- What do we need to know in order to implement supervision?

Step 2: the 'how' of implementation
- How are we going to find out what we need to know?

Step 3: the 'what now' of implementation
- Having determined what we need to know, how we are going to find out?
- What is our programme Now?

IMPLEMENTING SUPERVISION AT ORGANISATIONAL LEVEL

Here I offer the 3-Step method as simple guide to the implementation of supervision in an organisation. This section is an outline only, as a detailed plan falls outside the scope of this book. However, I hope it demonstrates the versatility and flexibility of the method. It offers a rough structure, outline or framework; however, the actual content of an implementation programme may vary greatly between organisations. The main point I wish to make is the need to do the homework. In my view it would be a pity to rush into clinical supervision without adequate thought and preparation beforehand, as that reduces the odds of its success and therefore wastes valuable resources.

The three steps are outlined in Box 10.2 and are discussed in more detail in the following section.

 THINKING POINT

If you were involved in implementing supervision in an organisation, what would you need to consider before you started and how would you go about implementing it?

Initially those charged with the implementation of clinical supervision will need to put their thinking caps on. It is also useful to contact other organisations that have already implemented supervision in order to learn from their experience.

Step 1: What do we need to know?

The implementation of clinical supervision requires a certain amount of thinking, assessment and decision-making. The 'What do we need to know?' question may be unpacked a bit into four sections: investigation, preparation, implementation and evaluation.

Investigation

- What is the purpose of supervision for the organisation?
- What are our goals and objectives?
- What is the situation of our organisation at the moment regarding those goals and objectives? In other words, what is the baseline?
- What supervision or similar activities are already taking place?

Preparation

- What training and preparation is needed?
- What skills and training have people already received?
- What expertise exists already amongst the workforce?
- What courses and other ways of preparing people are available in the area?
- What is the cost of these programmes?

Implementation

- What method of implementation will we use (across the board, start small, top-down, bottom-up, voluntary, compulsory, etc.)?
- What kind of supervision seems most desirable? (managerial, non-managerial, individual, team, group)?

Evaluation

- What do we need to measure in order to determine supervision's effectiveness or 'added value'?

There may already be a great deal of existing measures in place which might be expected to show an improvement, such as absenteeism, staff satisfaction surveys, client satisfaction surveys, etc.

Step 2: How are we going to find out what we need to know?

For most of the questions there are three main sources of information:

1. Published literature: books, articles, official documents, briefing papers, etc.
2. Other organisations.
3. The staff working for the organisation.

The staff working for the organisation are a great source of information which should not be underestimated. If people feel that they are consulted and that their views and opinions are taken into account, they are much more likely to be active participants in the process. The actual method of consultation will depend on what seems appropriate and will vary from organisation to organisation. A range of methods would seem a good idea to get a good all-round view.

Step 3: What Now is our programme of investigation, preparation, implementation and evaluation?

The main activities in this step are collating and categorising all the information generated in Step 2, before making decisions as to which actions will be taken. The 'how' step will have generated a great deal of information, which will now need to be collated and categorised. It is only when this has been done that decisions can be taken as to which actions seem most likely to be appropriate and effective.

Elsewhere I have written about the two main ways in which supervision in an organisation can be looked at: from the level of the organisation (the macro level), or from the level of the individuals working within it (the micro level). Both levels need to be taken into account when setting up a supervision programme, as what would seem to work well for the organisation may not be beneficial to the individuals and vice versa. (For a further discussion see van Ooijen 2000:144–154.)

I should just like to say that it would be great if a supervision programme could be implemented within a spirit of play and curiosity. We need to be aware of the danger of forming dogmatic ways of working, even if in the short term this may have the effect of helping to reduce uncertainty, but dogma kills creativity. I have noticed in myself that when my reflections seem to come too easily, this is a sure sign that a shake-up is needed!

Preparation is essential, but yet, despite all our spadework beforehand, we do not know how something is going to work until we actually do it. It would be a pity if implementation was done in a rigid 'This is how you do it' manner, as that is likely to be counter-productive. In my view, it needs to remain light, free and creative, as reflection cannot be forced and insights do not occur on demand. Although evaluation is important, it will not always be possible to have a specific outcome after a session. I find that frequently the penny does not drop until a few hours or even days after a session. Therefore it is good to encourage people to keep a journal, however brief, of new insights and perspectives. Although, clearly, such a journal belongs to the practitioner alone, it can be used by them as a source of outcomes and achievements, which could feed into both their own individual performance review process and the evaluation of the effectiveness of supervision – both theirs and that of the organisation. In other words, personal evidence can feed into organisational evidence.

CONCLUSION

In this chapter I first discussed some of the purposes of supervision as well as some thoughts on how it might usefully be implemented. There is more to supervision than monitoring people's performance. As stated elsewhere in the book, the quality of the relationship is key to the success of supervision, whether this is managerial or non-managerial. If the relationship is good, clinical supervision provided by the manager can work very well. For example, if learning needs are identified, the manager is in an ideal situation to make the relevant experience possible for the supervisee. Managerial supervision is not the same as individual performance review, as for supervision to work well it has to take place much more frequently than once or twice a year. However, supervision can perhaps be integrated with individual programme reviews, which might make it less of a one-off exercise which, to be honest, often gets forgotten about until the following year. Clinical supervision can also feed into any formal staff development programmes, courses or other developmental opportunities. In general, closer relationships between managers and their staff can only help to develop and improve relationships.

The people who work in an organisation should be seen as its greatest asset. It is therefore useful to involve people from all levels in the implementation of a supervision programme. It is good to work with groups of staff in order to discover how they see the organisation, its successes as well its failures. It is also good to ask them for their ideas for solutions, however wacky they may be. Good communications between all the levels in an organisation will minimise misunderstandings and create understanding and excitement. I stated above that clinical supervision could feed into other activities, such as individual performance review. However, this will only work if people feel they can be honest and that their opinions, creative ideas or ideas for more efficient ways of working do not pose a threat to their manager or colleagues. There needs to be an atmosphere of freedom and generosity; people need to feel that they can grow and develop, even if this means that eventually they outgrow the organisation and go elsewhere. An organisation with that kind of dynamic atmosphere will not have any problems in recruiting new people, as there will be a freedom from fear, encouragement of creativity, reward for success and help with areas that need further development.

Questions for further reflection

- Which type of supervision – managerial, non-managerial or a combination – do you feel is most appropriate for your situation?

- What are your reasons for this?

- How does your preferred type compare to what is in place in your situation at the moment?

- What might you want to do to change the way in which supervision is provided in your organisation?

- Who might be able to support you in this?

Conclusion

I am starting to write this conclusion while travelling on a train through the North East of the Netherlands. The sky is overcast, it is early evening and there is a hint of autumn in the air. I am Dutch born but have not lived here for a few decades, although I try to visit the country several times a year. Today I am on my way to visit one of my sisters who has moved a long way away (by Dutch standards) and I have not been to this part of the country for a very long time. The landscape surprises me, as it is much more varied than I expect.

It occurs to me that today's journey is a perfect metaphor for supervision. As the train guides me through the country of my birth, so in supervision we are guided or facilitated through our professional experience. Both journeys imply a return, an opportunity to take another look, to view the landscape from different angles, which creates a different view. It is not easy to do this by ourselves, we need someone to help us, to ask the naïve questions, to alert us to the fact that our view is not the only one. Perhaps a 'super' vision involves an awareness that there are many different visions, all of which are more or less valid, depending on our position. Supervision implies a willingness to let go of the tight hold we have over our own current vision and being open to let in some other possibilities. The effect is a view or vision that has expanded. From the train I view a landscape that has moved on since I was last here as a child. And yet, without too much imagination, I see the country of my childhood, the one I experienced and read about at school. Similarly, in supervision I do not lose my original position, rather it becomes one of several ways of looking at what I have brought. A supervisee who feels stuck in his work with a client, for example, does not necessarily feel miraculously unstuck as a result of supervision, although this can happen. Rather, the stuckness itself may have acquired a different meaning. It is even possible that the stuckness is seen as valuable in that it offers an opportunity to pay attention to whatever it is that is causing it.

So supervision may be seen as part of the journey of lifelong learning. I believe that the journey never stops. As I said in my earlier book, it can be dangerous to regard ourselves as an expert, if that means that we have nothing more to learn. Today's knowledge may tomorrow be regarded as quaint superstition. Also, the helping professions are concerned with people, who can always surprise us even when we think that we know everything. So, no matter how experienced we become I believe that supervision remains an important part of our work.

My aim for this book has been to provide a clear framework for all aspects of supervision. I want it to be easy to remember as well as flexible and adaptable so that it can be used in a wide variety of professional settings. As I stated in the Introduction, supervision is rapidly becoming an activity in its own right, with its own models, skills, methods and techniques.

I hope that this book offers a useful contribution.

References

Benner P, Wrubel J 1989 The primacy of caring, stress and coping in health and illness. Addison-Wesley, New York

Bollas C 1987 The shadow of the object. Psychoanalysis of the unthought known. Free Association Books, London

Bond T 2000 Standards and ethics for counselling in action, 2nd edn. Sage Publications, London

Bond M, Holland S 1998 Skills of clinical supervision for nurses. Open University Press, Buckingham

Bramley W 1996 The supervisory couple in broad-spectrum psychotherapy. Free Association Books, London

British Broadcasting Corporation 2002 The century of the self. BBC2 24 March

Carlowe J 1998 Value nurses and they will stay. Nursing Standard 12(27):12–13

Carroll M 1996 Counselling supervision. Theory, skills and practice. Cassell, London

Casement 1985 On learning from the patient. Tavistock, London

Castaneda C 1990 The teachings of Don Juan. A Yaqui way of knowledge. Arkana Books, London

Chakravarti A 1997 Teachings of Buddha. Rider, London

Covey S R 1992 The 7 habits of highly effective people. Simon and Schuster, London

Cutcliffe J R, Butterworth T, Proctor B (eds) 2001 Fundamental themes in clinical supervision. Routledge, London

Driscoll J 2000 Practising clinical supervision. A reflective approach. Baillière Tindall, Edinburgh

Driver C, Martin M 2002 Supervising psychotherapy. Sage Publications, London

Gilbert M C, Evans K 2000 Psychotherapy supervision. An integrative relational approach to psychotherapy supervision. Open University Press, Buckingham

Goss S, McLeod J 1999 Research news. Counselling 10(4):289

Guggenbuhl-Craig A 1996 Power in the helping professions. Spring Publications, Woodstock, CT

Hakesley-Brown R 2001/2 RCN magazine Winter: 1

Hawkins P, Shohet R 1989 Supervision in the helping professions, 1st edn. Open University Press, Buckingham

Hawkins P, Shohet R 2000 Supervision in the helping professions, 2nd edn. Open University Press, Buckingham

Hawley H 1993 Reawakening the spirit in work. The power of Dharmic management. Berrett-Koehler, San Francisco

Heider J 1992 The Tao of leadership. Wildwood House, Aldershot

Heimann P 1950 On countertransference. International Journal of Psychoanalysis 31:81–84

Heyward C 1994 When boundaries betray us. Beyond illusions of what is ethical in therapy and life. HarperCollins, San Francisco

Hobson RF 1985 Forms of feeling: the heart of psychotherapy. Tavistock Publications, London

Holloway E 1995 Clinical supervision. A systems approach. Sage Publications, Thousand Oaks, CA

Hycner R, Jacobs L 1995 The healing relationship in Gestalt therapy. A dialogic/self psychology approach. The Gestalt Journal Press, Highlands, NY

Inskipp F, Proctor B 1993 Making the most of supervision. The art, craft and tasks of counselling supervision, Part 1. Cascade Publications, Twickenham

Inskipp F, Proctor B 1995 Making the most of supervision, Part 2. Cascade Publications, Twickenham

Jacoby M 1995 Supervision and the interactive field. In: Kugler P (ed) Jungian perspectives on clinical supervision. Daimon, Einsiedeln, Switzerland

Jenkins P 2001 Supervisory responsibility and the law. In: Wheeler S, King D (eds) Supervising counsellors, issues of responsibility. Sage Publications, London, pp 22–24

Johns C 1997 Reflective practice and clinical supervision – part I: the reflective turn. European Nurse 2(2):87–97

Kell C 2002 Can counsellors adequately supervise non-counsellors? Counselling and Psychotherapy Journal 13(7):36–37

Klauser H A 1986 Writing on both sides of the brain. San Francisco: HarperCollins

Kugler P (ed) 1995 Jungian perspectives on clinical supervision. Daimon, Einsiedeln, Switzerland

Langs R 1994 Doing supervision and being supervised. Karnac Books, London

Larrabee M J (ed) 1993 An ethic of care. Feminist and intradisciplinary perspectives. Routledge, New York

Lomas P 2001 The limits of interpretation, revised edn. Robinson, London

Luria Z 1993 A methodological critique. In: Larrabee M J (ed) An ethic of care. Feminist and interdisciplinary perspectives. Routledge, New York

Mandler G 2000 A psychodynamic approach to brief therapy. Sage Publications, London

Moore N 1995 Michael Fordham's theory and practice of supervision. In: Kugler P (ed) Jungian perspectives on clinical supervision. Daimon, Einsiedeln, Switzerland

Noddings N 1986 Caring: a feminine approach to ethics and moral education. University of California Press, Berkeley

Page S, Wosket V 2001 Supervising the counsellor. A cyclical model, 2nd edn. Brunner-Routledge, Hove

Parsloe E 1999 The manager as coach and mentor, 2nd edn. Chartered Institute of Personnel and Development, London

Pirsig R 1978 Zen and the art of motorcycle maintenance. Corgi Books, London

Proctor B 2000 Group supervision. A guide to creative practice. Sage Publications, London

Rothschild B 2000 The body remembers. The psychopathology of trauma and trauma treatment. W W Norton, New York

Schore A N 2001 Minds in the making: attachment, the self-organising brain and developmentally-orientated psychoanalytic psychotherapy. British Journal of Psychotherapy 17(3):299–328

Steel C 2002 Wat is wijsheid? [what is wisdom?] Filosofie Magazine 11(5):30–32 (in Dutch)

Taylor K 1995 The ethics of caring. Hanford Mead Publishers, Santa Cruz

Thomas L 1998 Editorial. Nursing Standard 12(27):3

Tuckman B 1965 Developmental sequence in small groups. Psychological Bulletin 63:384–399

Usher C H, Borders L D 1993 Practising counsellors' preferences for supervisory style and emphasis. Counsellor Education and Supervision 33: 66–79

Vachon M 1996 What makes a team? Palliative Care Today 1:34–35 van Ooijen E 2000 Clinical supervision. A practical guide. Churchill Livingstone, Edinburgh

van Ooijen E, Charnock A 1994 Sexuality and patient care. A guide for nurses and teachers. Chapman & Hall, London

Watson J 1988 Nursing: human science and human care. A theory of nursing. National League for Nursing, New York

Webb A, Wheeler S 1998 How honest do counsellors dare to be in the supervisory relationship. An exploratory study. British Journal of Guidance and Counselling 26:509–524

Williams S, Michie S, Pattani S 1998 Improving the health of the NHS workforce. Report of the partnership on the health of the NHS workforce. Nuffield Trust, London

Wood M 2002 Start thinking. London Review of Books 24(5):10–11

Appendix: Organisations and journals

SUPERVISION IN EUROPE

The Association of National Organisations for Supervision in Europe (ANSE) is a useful resource for accessing information on local member associations, supervisors or training. They may be contacted through:
Louis van Kessel, c/o Boeslaan 19,
NL-6703 EN Wageningen, The Netherlands
Tel: +31-317-423259
Fax: +31-317-422267
E-mail: anse-info@supervision-eu.org
Website: http://www.supervision-eu.org/anse

Centre for Staff Team Development,
c/o Bath Consultancy Group,
24 Gay Street, Bath BA1 2PD
Website: http://bathconsultancygroup.com

SUPERVISION JOURNALS

Supervisie in Opleiding en Beroep Tijdschrift voor Professioneel Begeleiden [Supervision in Training and in the Professions. Research News for Professional Support]
ISSN 0920-2404
Bohn Stafleu Van Loghum, Postbus 246,
NL-3990 GA Houten, The Netherlands
Tel: +31-30-6385700
Fax: +31-30-6395839
E-mail: klantenservice@bsl.nl
Website: http://www.bsl.nl

Forum Supervision
ISSN 0942-0045246
Verlag Edition Diskord, Schwärzlocher Str. 104/b,
D-72070 Tübingen, Germany
Tel: +49-7071-40102
Fax: +49-7071-44710

Freie Assoziation [Free Association]
ISSN 1434-7849
Daedalus Verlag Joachim Herbst, Oderstraße 25,
D-48145 Münster, Germany
Tel: +49-251-231355
E-mail: info@daedalus-verlag.de
Website: http://www.freie-assoziation.de

Supervision: Zeitschrift für berufsbezogene Beratung [Supervision. Journal for Professionally Oriented Support]
ISSN 1431-7168
Votum Verlag GmbH., Grevener Straße 89–91,
D-48159 Münster, Germany
Tel: +49-251-265140
Fax: +49-251-2651420
E-mail: info@votum-verlag.de
Website: http://www.votum-verlag.de

OSC – Organisationsberatung, Supervision, Coaching [OSC – Organisational Support, Supervision, Coaching]
ISSN 0946-9834
Verlag Leske & Budrich, Postfach 300 551,
D-51334 Leverkusen, Germany
Tel: +49-2171-49070
E-mail: lesbudpubl@aol.com
Website: http://www.leske-budrich.de

Profile. Internationale Zeitschrift für Veränderung, Lernen, Dialog [Profile. International Journal for Change, Learning, Dialogue]

ISSN 1615-5084
Tel: +49-221-5304411
Fax: +49-221-5302062
E-mail: info@ehp-koeln.com
Website: http://www.ehp-koeln.com

The Clinical Supervisor. The Journal of Supervision in Psychotherapy and Mental Health

The Haworth Press, 10 Alice Street, Binghamton,
NY 13904-1580, USA
Tel: +1-800-607-722-5857
Fax: +1-800-895-0582
E-mail: getinfo@haworthpressinc.com
Website: http://www.haworthpressinc.com

FEEDBACK REQUEST

I should be very interested in any feedback you may have on this book. Suggestions for alterations, inclusions in later editions or ideas for further publications would also be gratefully received.

Any comments should be sent to:

Els van Ooijen
Nepenthe Consultancy
5 Normanton Road
Clifton, Bristol BS8 2TY, UK
Tel: +44-117-908-9143

Index